Chapter titles

Using this book

This book is meant to be helpful to everyone who finds themselves being asked to plan or evaluate an activity intended to promote healthier eating.

It is intended to be read at three levels:

1   You can just read the text ignoring all the boxes. This should give you a basic understanding of how to collect and use information for planning, monitoring and evaluating and what problems you might encounter.

2   If you want to find out a little more about some subject then you will find it explained in more detail in the boxes. The text will indicate which boxes you should look at to find out more about each subject.

3   If you want to take the subject further you will find suggested reading at the end of each chapter.

At frequent intervals in the book you will find suggestions that you go and talk to people with expert knowledge. You are strongly urged to take this advice. It will save you wasting hours of time and money and may make the difference between success and failure.

List of boxes, figures and tables

Chapter 1 – The need for information – Planning, Monitoring and Evaluation

Chapter 2 – What information to collect

Chapter 3 – Planning the study – Writing the protocol

Chapter 4 – Study design for monitoring and evaluation

Chapter 5 – What is meant by validation

Chapter 10 – Measurement of attitudes

Chapter 11 – Methods for studying habitual food consumption and eating patterns (food frequency questionnaires and diet history)

Chapter 12 – Methods for studying food consumption (specified time methods) – by A. Bone

Chapter 13 – Estimating nutrient intake

Chapter 14 – Measuring food consumption – trends in retail food sales and food purchase – by M. Clapham and N. J. G. Field

Chapter 16 – Presenting the results – by T. Marshall

Foreword

For almost six million years, humans have wandered the earth as nomadic beings, surviving nutritionally on what was available to them, mostly vegetarian, together with occasional animals that were caught. Over the last five thousand years, and, particularly over the last hundred years, and more especially in recent times, our diet has changed dramatically, with the advent of mass production techniques, convenience foods, additives, colourings, etc. There is an increasing belief that our modern diet may be, at least, in part, responsible for some of the more common diseases which now beset mankind.

To be able to objectively assess people's precise eating habits, is extremely difficult. This book is a very real attempt, for the first time, to provide a guide to those who work in the nutrition survey field and represents a collaborative effort by Dr. John Kemm, Professor David Booth and their colleagues, Tim Marshall, Neil Field, Alison Bone and Mike Clapham. It should prove to be an invaluable guide to health promoters and others in the field of influencing healthy eating.

The Nutritional Advisory Group of the West Midlands Regional Health Authority have supported the tremendous effort to produce this book of Dr. Kemm and Professor Booth with finance and in many other ways.

Bernard J. Smits, KSG, MB, BS, FRCP
Consultant Physician/Gastroenterologist
Chairman, West Midlands Regional Nutrition Advisory Group

1 · The need for information: Planning, Monitoring and Evaluation

Summary

Information is needed at three places in the planning and running of any healthy eating promotion, before it starts, while it is running and at the end. Background information is needed to ensure that the nutritional and health promotion theory underlying any promotion of healthier eating is sound. Information is needed before the start to select target groups, to set objectives and to choose suitable methods of health promotion. Information is then needed during the programme to check how things are going and after the programme to see how things have changed.

Evaluation provides evidence of the usefulness of a programme and its components. Evaluation is used first to develop the programme (formative evaluation) and then to assess its overall effect (summative evaluation).

Introduction

To monitor means to keep under observation or to measure at intervals. To evaluate means to use the results of monitoring to obtain evidence of the value (i.e. effect) of an activity such as a promotion of healthier eating. This first chapter explains why monitoring what people are eating and what they think and feel about food is important. The rest of the book is about the various ways in which you can collect and use this information in your region, district or town.

The use of information

Collecting information is an essential part of any health promotion activity. The information needed is summarised in Table 1.1. Figure 1.1 shows some of the steps involved in a programme intended to influence what people eat or what they think about food. It can be seen that information is needed at three stages. First, information is needed at the planning stage in order to decide what the programme should do and how to do it. Once the programme is under way, information is needed again to see how it is going and whether it needs to be altered in any way.

Finally when the programme is established (or completed) information has to be collected in order to show how or if things have changed. This taken with other information can provide evidence on how successful the programme has been and provide a basis for the decision whether the programme or a part of it should be continued (or repeated).

Table 1.1   Information needs for promotion of healthier eating

Theoretical base for link between food and health
Food consumption and habits
Sources of information about food
Practical and cultural constraints on food availability
Other characteristics of target group
How and why these things change

(This list is expanded in Box 2.1)

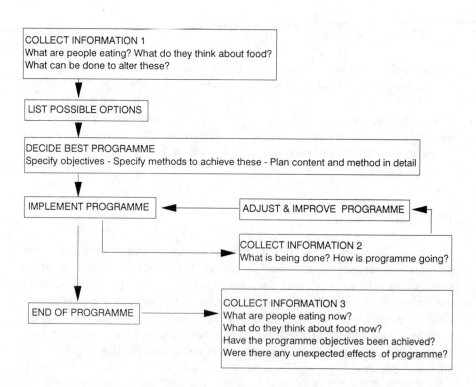

Fig 1.1   Planning cycle for promotion of healthier eating

Summary of dietary recommendations from the NACNE 1983 report

These recommendations are long term targets for the average national per capita intake. Intermediate targets are shown in brackets. It is recommended that individual intakes should be changed to bring the national average towards these targets.

1 *Energy*
   Maintain optimal body weight for height and sex by adjusting energy intake and increasing amount of exercise.

2 *Fat*
   Decrease total fat from 38% to 30% (34%) of total energy intake.
   Decrease saturated fatty acids from 18% to 10% (15%) of total energy intake.
   No specific recommendation on unsaturated fatty acids but previous two recommendations will ensure increase in P/S ratio from about 0.24 to 0.44.

3 *Fibre*
   Increase dietary fibre from 20 g/day to 30 g/day (25 g/day)

4 *Sucrose*
   Decrease sucrose intake from 38 kg/yr to 20 kg/yr (34 kg/yr)

5 *Salt*
   Decrease salt intake by 3 g (1 g) per day

6 *Alcohol*
   Decrease alcohol intake from 6% to 4% (5%) of total energy intake.

NOTE The starting levels quoted were the estimated situation in 1980.

Healthier eating – the underlying theories are important

Health promoters wish to influence people to take up 'healthier eating'. It is known that people who eat in certain ways have a reduced risk of developing heart disease and other illnesses. The expert consensus is that there is now sufficient evidence to justify action. The National Advisory Committee on Nutrition Education (NACNE) suggested what they considered to be a

---

Box 1.2

Types of evidence which support links between an eating pattern and health or disease

1   *Epidemiological evidence of association*
    Showing particular eating patterns and disease frequency vary together
    between countries or different groups within countries.
    Comparison between countries or different groups within countries.
    Studies of secular trends (changes over time).
    Comparison of migrant populations and populations in country of origin.
    Case control studies (compare foods eaten by people with and without the
    disease).
    Cohort studies (compare disease frequency in people with different food
    intakes).

2   *Disease models in animals*
    Showing disease can be induced in experimental animals by subjecting
    them to suspect eating pattern.

3   *Biochemical and physiological studies*
    Demonstrating possible mechanisms by which eating pattern could cause
    disease.

4   *Clinical studies*
    Showing that changes in the eating pattern affect the disease process
    and/or chances of recurrence.

5   *Population intervention studies*
    Showing that when eating patterns are altered in the desired direction the
    disease frequency is reduced.

    (This last is much the strongest type of evidence but in most cases is not
    available.)

'healthier' eating pattern (Box 1.1). Similar but slightly different recommendations have been made by other committees (Box 9.5). Most promotion of 'healthier' eating (in developed countries) is based on the findings of such committees.

The underlying reason for attempting to influence people's eating patterns is some nutritional theory that changing their eating pattern in a particular way will improve their health. If we did not have a theory that eating habits affected

4

health, there would be no reason for trying to change eating habits. For example, the reason for encouraging people to eat more dietary fibre or to eat less saturated fats is the belief based on epidemiological, clinical and experimental findings that this would improve their health. If our beliefs about the effect of eating habits were wrong then changing these eating habits would not improve health. The underlying nutritional theory in health promotion does matter: an enthusiastic intention to promote health is not enough.

Box 1.2 shows the types of evidence that support theories of healthier eating. The weight of evidence supports the view that current advice on healthy eating is broadly correct. Nonetheless health promoters have given different advice in the past. Only fifteen years ago most doctors, dieticians and health educators were advising people to eat generous amounts of meat and full fat dairy products and to avoid starchy foods because they were 'fattening'. These earlier theories on the links between food and health have later been shown to be wrong. As more evidence is collected we may have to change or tighten up the details of what we now recommend as healthier eating. However while current eating patterns persist the main messages are unlikely to change.

This book will not examine the evidence for the nutritional theories which undertake healthier eating advice nor consider how to assess them. However, promoters of healthier eating must keep an eye on expert consensus to check that the scientific basis for their work is still sound. When planning or assessing a healthy eating programme one of the questions should be 'is the nutritional theory correct?'.

Any programme to promote healthier eating should therefore always be designed in consultation with a well informed dietician or nutritionist. They will know the current consensus of expert thinking on the details of nutritional recommendations and how they are best interpreted. Examples of some more recent developments which might be taken into account are shown in Box 1.3.

Activities intended to promote healthier eating are also based on theories of how people's eating behaviour can be changed. These theories describe what knowledge, beliefs, motives, feelings and opportunities influence eating choices and how these influences can be affected. Sound social, psychological and educational theory is also essential to effective health promotion. When planning your programmes you will also want to consult people with these expertises.

Setting healthier eating objectives

A key part of planning any healthier eating programme is setting the objectives. This means stating exactly what you hope to achieve by the programme and exactly what you hope to change. Objectives are sometimes stated in vague terms such as 'increase the number of people eating wholemeal bread', 'encourage people to eat more dietary fibre' or 'increase awareness of the link between fat consumption and heart disease'. At other times objectives are stated in quantitative terms such as 'By 1995 60% of the population will eat mostly wholemeal bread' or 'At the end of the programme 80% of the school will be able to name five foods which are good sources of dietary fibre'. Some more examples of healthier eating objectives are given in Box 1.4. The way the objectives are set will suggest the types of information which should be used to monitor the programme.

Box 1.4

Examples of healthier eating objectives

Targets from Oxford regional health promotion plan

1   To increase the proportion of those aged 18-64 who eat wholemeal bread
    most of the time from 40% in 1986 to 50% in 1994.

2   To increase the proportion of those in social class IIIM, IV and V aged
    18-64 who eat wholemeal bread most of the time from about 30% in 1986
    to 45% in 1994.

3   To increase the proportion of people aged 18-64 who used skimmed or
    semi-skimmed milk most of the time from 27% in 1986 to 40% in 1994.

4   To increase the proportion of those in social class IIIM, IV and V aged
    18-64 who use skimmed or semi-skimmed milk most of the time from
    about 22% in 1986 to about 38% in 1994.

(Note the very precise quantitively stated objectives and the targeting with the
intention of reducing social class inequalities.)

Source: *Health For All in the Oxford Region* – A Health Promotion Review 1987.
        Publ. Oxford RHA.

Targeting groups

So far we have talked about 'people' as though they were all the same but of
course this is not so. Within any region, district or town there will be many
different groups. People can be divided into groups on the basis of many characteristics such as age, sex and ethnic group. Other important characteristics on
which people may be grouped are shown in Box 1.5.

Different groups may have different eating habits. Young people tend to have
different eating patterns from old age pensioners. A family recently arrived
from Bangladesh eats very different foods from an indigenous family. Higher
income families eat more wholemeal bread, more fresh fruit and more fresh
meat than lower income families. Other examples of how eating habits differ
between income groups are shown in Box 1.6.

Most health promotion policies include as one of their aims equity, the
reduction of differences in health between groups by improving the health of the

least advantaged. When we look at any population we will find some groups who have relatively healthy eating habits and some who do not. Groups with the least healthy eating patterns may be selected as targets for promotion of healthier eating. Unless we have information on the differences between groups we cannot promote equity.

Information on differences between groups is also needed if we are to use scarce health promotion resources most effectively. Concentrating health promotion effort on the groups with the least healthy habits may allow us to have the maximum effect on the health of the population. Furthermore any programme intended to reach everyone is unlikely to be successful because people differ in interests, lifestyles and the things that influence them.

Once the programme is underway we still need information on different groups. It is likely that some groups will respond to the programme while others will not.

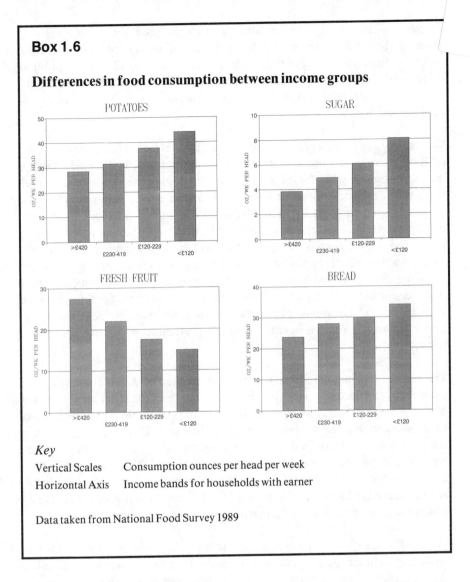

Box 1.6

Differences in food consumption between income groups

POTATOES

SUGAR

FRESH FRUIT

BREAD

Key

Vertical Scales   Consumption ounces per head per week

Horizontal Axis   Income bands for households with earner

Data taken from National Food Survey 1989

For example many programmes which included increased use of semi-skimmed milk among their aims found that women were more likely to respond than men. If we can identify the groups in which the programme is failing we can try to adjust the programme to make it work better in these groups. At the end of the programme we want to know not only its overall success but also any differences in its success between groups. We can then use this knowledge to design better programmes in the future.

Choosing objectives and methods

Information on target groups is essential if we are to set proper objectives and choose the best methods for promotion of healthier eating. If the target group

9

already has the eating habits or attitudes that the programme is intended to promote the effort is wasted. If the attitudes and eating habits of the target group are too different from those that the programme is intended to promote the messages will seem irrelevant and the programme will fail. We have to know where people are starting from in order to set sensible objectives for promotion of healthier eating.

We also need to know a great deal about the things which affect people's choice of food in order to choose methods of promotion which will work. Groups differ not only in what food they eat but also in what they know about food, what they feel about food and the situations in which they eat. The food knowledge of a group of dieticians will be very different from that of a group of unemployed school leavers. A school child from the indigenous community may prefer foods which could be repulsive to his Hindu or Islamic classmate. The food choices available to a person with a car and high income are very different from the choices available to an unemployed person without transport and a poor command of English. These differences between groups in food knowledge, feelings about food, access to food and uses of foods are just as important to designing a healthier eating programme as differences in food consumption.

The recent programme to prevent rickets in children of Asian origin is a good example of the need to match the promotion methods to the target group. The advice given to parents of white children (ensure your childrens' skin is exposed to the sun and that the child eats foods rich in vitamin D such as liver and fatty fish) was not acceptable to the Asian target group and the styles of most of the posters and pamphlets were not culturally relevant. The messages and the approach had to be redesigned to take account of foods which normally featured in the Asian diet and of beliefs about decency in dress so as to make the programme acceptable and meaningful to the Asian community.

We need to identify blocks to healthier eating. There is little point in advising women in an inner city estate to buy wholemeal bread and semi-skimmed milk if the local shops do not stock these items. In this example any programme which did not include measures to improve the availability of these products would be futile.

This section has shown the need for accurate information in order to plan effective promotion of healthier eating.

Working with food retailers and suppliers

Promotion of healthier eating very often involves increasing the availability of healthier food choices and therefore working with food retailers or suppliers. Information is also the key to success here. Retailers will be interested in what the demand for new food lines is likely to be and which other retailers already stock these lines. The amount of any food line sold will be affected by price, location in shop (is it highly visible?) and perhaps advertising, as well as customer interest cultivated by the media or by local health promotion activity. Restaurant and snack bar owners and canteen managers will want the same sort of information before agreeing to add new items to the menu. Information is as important for health promotion through increasing availability of healthier choices as it is for health promotion through altering consumers' knowledge and attitudes.

What is evaluation?

Using information to improve or to assess the effectiveness of programmes is usually called evaluation. Evaluation is more than monitoring because it is concerned not only to record what things are changing but also to assess to what extent the health promotion activity was responsible for causing those changes.

There are two main types of evaluation, formative evaluation and summative evaluation. Formative evaluation involves collecting information while the programme is running and using it to develop and improve the programme. Summative evaluation involves collecting information about an established (or completed) programme in order to decide whether it should be continued (or repeated). Summative evaluation is discussed more fully in the next section. If you have been asked to perform an evaluation you should be clear whether it is a formative or summative evaluation or a mixture of both which is required.

Evaluations may also be divided into process evaluations and outcome evaluations. The meaning of these terms and their relation to formative and summative evaluation is discussed in Chapter 8. Evaluation may involve many different methods of collecting information. The methods chosen and the information collected will largely depend on what type of evaluation is required. More information on evaluation methods is shown in Box 1.7.

In any evaluation three roles can be distinguished: the programme manager who will make decisions about the fate of the programme, the programme worker who is carrying out the programme and the evaluator. The evaluator has to be trusted and believed by both manager and worker. If trust breaks down the workers may feel that the evaluator does not understand what they are trying to achieve and is only being used by management to find an excuse to close the programme down. Alternatively the managers may feel that the evaluator is too closely identified with the programme worker and is just trying to justify continuing someone's pet project.

These difficulties are most likely to be avoided if everyone is agreed as to what the programme is trying to achieve and the methods of evaluation used are relevant and scientifically sound. Also you need to agree with both manager and workers before you start the evaluation how the information you collect should be used. An evaluator's life is not an easy one.

Box 1.7

Comparison of formative and summative evaluation

FORMATIVE EVALUATION	SUMMATIVE EVALUATION
Principal Question	
How is the programme going? How could it be adjusted to make it go better?	Did the programme achieve its objectives? Were there any unexpected effects? Is the programme worth repeating/continuing?
Main user of evaluation	
Programme staff	Programme managers
Main areas of enquiry	
Programme activities (process) e.g. Number of enquiries received, leaflets issued, attendance at events, etc.	Programme outcomes e.g. Number of people eating wholemeal bread, number believing they can reduce their risk of heart disease, etc.
Feelings of staff and public about programme.	Feelings of public about healthier eating.
Main methods of enquiry	
Study of programme activity records. Observation of activities.	Surveys of eating behaviour, beliefs, etc., compared with prior or control data.
Interviews with staff and public.	Interviews with staff and public.

NOTE

In practice there is usually considerable overlap between these two types of evaluation and most evaluations will have some of the characteristics of both types.

Ideally the evaluator should be independent of manager and worker but in practice the evaluator's role is often combined with that of the manager or of the worker. In these circumstances the information collected may be considered less reliable and if you are evaluating your own project you will have to be especially sure that the methods you use to collect and analyse information can be defended.

Value for money – summative evaluation of healthier eating promotion

At a time when money and other resources are short and with the new culture of purchaser-provider relationships in the NHS it is particularly important to ensure that every activity is worthwhile. Managers quite rightly look at healthier eating promotion activities and ask the questions 'What is this activity achieving? Could the resources used be better used for some other purpose?' In other words they want a summative evaluation.

Methods of evaluation ought to be decided when the programme is being planned but all too often this does not happen and one has to try and add an evaluation onto a programme which is already running.

The first task for the evaluator is to agree what were the objectives of the programme, that is what it was intended to achieve. If you are lucky these will be clearly written down but very often they are only vague ideas in someone's head. When the objectives are agreed you can try and devise methods to test whether they have been achieved or not.

The programme may also have had unintended effects good or bad. The evaluator needs to think what these might have been and devise methods to test whether they occurred.

The evaluator will need to describe what activities have taken place in the programme. How did the programme staff spend their time? What meetings were held, what film, leaflets and posters were used and so on? This information is needed to assess whether the programme was carried out as intended and what resources were actually used.

Ways of collecting the different types of information are described in later chapters of this book. (Chapter 8 – Describing what was done; Chapter 9 – Measuring Knowledge; Chapter 10 – Measuring Attitudes; Chapters 11-13 – Measuring Consumption; Chapter 14 – Measuring Availability).

All this information can then be used to decide what has changed while the programme was running and what resources have been used. The final step in evaluation is to decide to what extent the programme should be credited with causing any changes that were observed. Chapter 4 discusses the different ways of doing this. If the programme's achievements were not as expected it may be possible to decide why this was so. It may also be possible to identify which parts of the programme worked best or see ways of improving the programme.

Information is collected to be used

The information you collect will be of little use unless you write a clear and accurate report of your findings. This report must then be distributed to the people who should be interested in your results. Chapter 16 is about how to write reports in a way that enables people to understand what you have done and make the best use of your results.

The emphasis throughout this chapter has been on using information. The only reason for collecting information is to use it and if you are not sure how the information could be useful don't collect it.

Further Reading

Planning promotion of healthier eating activities

Ewles L. & Simnett I. (1985).
  Chapter 7 in Promoting Health: a Practical Guide to Health Education.
  Wiley, New York.
Green L. W., Kreater M. W., Deeds S. G. & Partridge K. B. (1980).
  Health Education Planning – A diagnostic approach. Mayfield Publishing,
  Palo Alto.
W.H.O. (1988).
  Education for health. A manual on health education in primary health care.
  W.H.O. Geneva. Chap. 3 Planning for health education in primary health care.
  (Focus on third world practice but good exposition of basic principles.)

Evidence for healthy eating theories

Doll R. & Peto R. (1981).
  The causes of cancer. Oxford University Press, Oxford.
Lewis B. (1980). 'Dietary prevention of ischaemic heart disease – a policy for the 80's'.
  British Medical Journal ii, 177-180.

Objectives for health promotion activities

St. Pierre R. G. (1982). 'Specifying outcomes in nutrition education evaluation.'
  Journal of Nutrition Education 14, 49-51.

Evaluation

Mullen P. D. & Ivenson D. (1982). Qualitative methods for evaluative research in
  health education programmes.
  Health Education (May/June) 11-18.
Herman J. L., Morris J. L. & Fitz-Gibbons C. T. (1987).
  Evaluators handbook. Sage Publications, California & London.

Nutbeam D., Smith C. & Catford J. (1990). Evaluation in health education.
A review of progress and possibilities.
Journal of Epidemiology and Community Health 44, 83-89.

Dietary targets

Select Committee on Nutrition and Human Needs. U.S. Senate (1977).
Dietary Goals for the U.S.A. (McGovan Report). U.S. Govt. Printing
Office 052-070-04376-8.

2 · What information to collect

Summary

This chapter lists the various types of information relevant to eating which you might consider collecting. These include awareness of food and health issues, knowledge, skills and behaviour related to eating and availability of food choices. There is a short discussion of the reasons why you might want to collect information in each of these areas. You must be selective and choose relatively few types of information to collect and then focus the items on your monitoring or evaluation.

> 'If you can count it, it doesn't count.
> If it counts, you can't count it.'
>
> Anon

Introduction

After you have decided that you are going to collect some information on what people are eating or what they think about food the next thing to decide is precisely what information you are going to collect. Box 2.1 gives a list of some of the information you might try to collect. The rest of the chapter discusses the advantages and disadvantages of collecting each type of information.

Beware of being too ambitious. If you try and collect too many pieces of information the whole study will become unmanageable and you may well end up with nothing. Select out of the list just those items that will be most useful.

What worries people about food

One of the aims of health promotion is often to 'empower' people, that is to increase their control over their own lives by increasing the number of choices available to them and their ability to choose. If we take this seriously it follows that we should not be deciding what people's problems are but instead asking them to decide what their problems are. Of course we may not agree about what is a problem or what is a solution but we are unlikely to do effective health promotion unless we are aware of and acknowledge the client's worries and hopes. We therefore need to know what people view as problems and as opportunities.

This information could be gathered by asking people to talk about what they felt

---
Box 2.1

**Items of information you might consider collecting
(the study variables)**

Awareness and agenda
1   Perceived problems – what are people's worries about food?
2   Awareness of nutrition and health issues

Knowledge and skills
3   Knowledge of links between food choices and health
4   Knowledge of what is in food
5   Cooking and shopping skills

Values
6   Cultural differences in what people want to eat
7   What people say they value about healthier eating
8   Perceived credibility of sources of information – whom do people trust?
9   Role models – whom do people wish to be like.

Behaviour
10 Meal patterns
11 Special diets
12 Frequency of consumption of different foods – how much – how often?
13 Intake of nutrients (energy, protein, fat, vitamins, minerals, etc.)
14 Shopping and cooking habits
15 Weight and weight control efforts

Availability
16 What foods are available in local shops – what price – how visible are
    they?
17 What is sold in restaurants, canteens, etc.

Background data
18 Age, sex, ethnicity, occupation, social class, income group, place of
    residence, etc. (see Box 1.5)

---

to be problems with eating, either in group discussions or in individual
interviews. An alternative would be to present people with a long list of possible
problems and ask them which of those things bothered them. One such possible
list is shown in Box 2.2 and an example of a questionnaire in Box 2.7. This
approach has the disadvantage that by including things in the list we are
suggesting that they might be a problem and by omitting things we are

Box 2.2

Possible worries about food

The NACNE Agenda
1 Fat content of food and types of fat
2 Fibre content of food
3 Refined sugars in food
4 Salt in food

The Food Hygiene Agenda
1 Bacterial food poisoning (Salmonella, Staphylocci, Botulism, Campylobacter, Listeria, etc.)
2 Contaminants (pesticides, vermin, foreign bodies)
3 Natural toxins

The Health Food Agenda
1 Additives & E numbers (colours, preservatives, antoxidants, etc.)
2 Organic and natural food
3 Irradiation
4 'Allergies'

The Disease Prevention Agenda
Heart disease, hypertension
Cancer, bowel disease
Arthritis, hyperactivity
Osteomalacia
Asthma and eczema etc.

The Wartime Agenda
1 Enough to eat
2 Enough fat and protein
3 Enough vitamins
4 Enough minerals

The Consumerist Agenda
1 Value for money – cost
2 Proper labelling
3 Adulteration with inferior substitutes
4 Water in food
5 Validity of health claims

The Ecological Agenda
1 Factory farming (kindness to animals, etc.)
2 Nitrate pollution
3 Exploitation of workers in food industry
4 Food packaging (energy costs, refuse etc.)

Spiritual Agendas
Is food Kosher, Hallal, I-tal, etc?
Vegetarianism

The Slimming Agenda

suggesting that we have not thought of them as possible problems. Different ways of asking questions are discussed further in Chapter 5.

Awareness

Before starting a health promotion activity we need to know how aware people are of the problems and of the possibilities of doing something about them.

People are unlikely to do anything about a health problem deliberately unless they are aware of its existence and the ways of solving it. 'Raising awareness' in food consumers, food providers or both is often stated as one of the objectives of a healthier eating promotion activity. It is necessary to measure awareness in the target population before and after the activity in order to see whether such an objective has been achieved.

Knowledge and beliefs

Increasing peoples' knowledge of the likely links between health and eating or their knowledge of what is in different foods (e.g. their nutrient content) is often an important component of healthier eating promotion though probably not the most important one. If a person does not know the eating habits which increase their risk of heart disease, how can they avoid them? How can someone set about choosing a high fibre diet if they don't know which foods are good sources of fibre? In planning a health promotion activity we therefore need to find out how much people know about the problem and its solutions. If we are trying to increase knowledge we need to measure it before and after the educational activity to see how far we have progressed towards our objective.

Everyone who has ever marked an exam (and most people who have taken one) will realise that knowledge is not easy to measure.

The first problem in measuring knowledge is to agree what information is correct which may be very difficult when talking about the links between food and health. Then we have to decide what areas of knowledge are most important to enable healthy eating choices and therefore ought to be tested. Lastly, we have to devise ways of finding out whether people know and understand that information in a way that they can act on. We have to do better than ask useless questions like 'Chips are bad for you – True or False?'. What knowledge to measure and how to do it is considered further in Chapter 9.

Skills

Lack of skills in menu-choosing shopping and cooking can limit people's ability to choose a healthy eating pattern. People who are not confident that they can make a nice meal starting from raw ingredients are likely to be restricted to foods which are highly processed or even ready prepared. These foods are likely to be more expensive and may have higher salt, fat and sugar contents than home prepared foods. Information on what skills people have may be very useful in planning or evaluating a healthier eating promotion.

Values

The reasons why any individual decides to eat one food rather than another are

20

very complex. Health considerations probably play only a very small part in what most people choose to eat. We are more likely to be able to influence eating patterns if we understand some of the values and beliefs that affect food choices and how the balance of motivation varies across people.

Very often health promoters must try to work with clients who come from a different cultural background to their own. They have very little chance of influencing eating patterns unless they understand the attitudes to food in their client's culture. Health promotion which conflicts with deeply held cultural values is almost certain to fail and likely to harm relations with the client.

It is obvious that attitudes to food differ considerably between ethnic and religious groups. We would expect a family from Bangladesh, a family from North India and an indigenous English family to prefer different foods.

Similarly most people know that the Islamic, Hindu and Jewish faiths have different laws as to what foods may be eaten. Chapter 15 gives further information on different ethnic groups. However, differences between groups within the same ethnic or religious communities are no less important.

The health promotion strategy has to be tailored so that it does not directly conflict with deeply held cultural values or beliefs. One study showed how women in the Welsh valleys had very firm ideas about what constituted a 'proper meal' and any healthier eating promotion which challenged those ideas would be strongly resisted. Similarly spending time in the evening in the pub or club drinking and perhaps eating is a deeply rooted tradition for some people; for them a strategy of making it possible to choose healthier pub food would probably be more successful than attempting to encourage a different style of eating.

Another attitude which will have a big effect on the success of a healthier eating promotion activity is what sources of information people trust. Health promotion messages may come from newspapers, radio, TV, food manufacturers, nurses, health visitors, health education officers, dieticians, general practitioners, hospital doctors, social workers, teachers, friends, relations and many other sources. We need to know which of these sources people listen to, believe and act upon (really value) so that we can choose the most effective way of putting the message across.

There are other values that we may wish to change. Are people fatalistic about the inevitability of heart disease? Do they think of low fat foods as boring and unappetising? Do they think that healthier eating is just another attempt by 'them' to stop us enjoying ourselves? Are they only really concerned to have a hearty meal or only really concerned to be slimmer? It will be essential to have information on the values and beliefs of the target group before planning a healthier eating promotion activity. If we are trying to change values we will need to measure them before and after in order to find out if we have succeeded. You will find more about how to measure values in Chapter 10.

Meal patterns

The times of day at which people usually eat, the sorts of meals they take (snacks, sit-down meals, etc.), the circumstances in which they eat them and where they eat are all useful in planning healthy eating promotion activity. Sometimes the eating pattern is the main focus of health promotion for example avoiding frequent eating of sugar containing snacks that leave sugar on the teeth. Information on the meal pattern is needed to make healthier eating messages relevant. Messages, based on three regular meals a day may prove to be totally inappropriate for many target groups.

Frequency of consumption of different foods

A change in how often people eat certain types of foods is usually one of the objectives of healthier eating promotion activity. Frequent consumption of traditional snack foods such as crisps, biscuits and sweets will tend to raise fat intake. Infrequent consumption of fruit and vegetables may result in low vitamin intake.

What foods are people eating? How often are they eating them? In what quantities are they eating them? These may all be important questions for planning or evaluating an activity intended to promote healthier eating.

However, you cannot ask about every food available and you must select relatively few foods to ask about. If the objective was to increase or decrease consumption of certain foods then obviously you will only be interested in broad categories of food (green vegetables, fat meat, etc.). If a researcher was interested in something as specific as fatty acid intake or additives they would have to specify the food in great detail (exact description of food and brand name). You will find more about the ways in which this sort of information can be collected in Chapters 11 and 12.

Measuring nutrient intake

Often the objectives of healthier eating are expressed in nutrient terms such as 'to increase consumption of dietary fibre and to decrease consumption of fat, refined sugars and salt'. Evaluation of such objectives must include some attempt to estimate consumption of those foods which are major sources of the nutrient in which we are interested. Surveys often ask about wholemeal bread because bread accounts for a large part of people's insoluble fibre intake and wholemeal bread contains more fibre than white bread. It is hoped that if people are changing from white to wholemeal bread for health reasons they will be increasing their consumption of fibre from bread and perhaps from other sources.

Questions are often asked about skimmed and semi-skimmed milk for similar reasons. If people are changing to fat reduced milks for health reasons then they might also be reducing other sources of fat in their diets.

Deciding which few foods to ask about when trying to estimate nutrient intake is very difficult. There has been little research on how food choice habits affect overall nutrient intake. Estimates of nutrient intake based on consumption of a few foods will be very crude though perhaps better than no estimates at all.

Sometimes it may be felt worthwhile to try and estimate nutrient intake by asking about a very wide range of foods. This avoids the problem of relying on a very few selected foods but is time consuming and introduces a host of new problems. You will find a much longer discussion of how to measure nutrient intake in Chapter 13.

Shopping and cooking arrangements

Where people buy food, how often they go food shopping (a big weekly shop or just before they want to eat the food) and who does the shopping are all useful things to know for promotion of healthier eating.

It is also helpful to know what cooking and food storage facilities people have. Is someone cooking on a single ring in a bed-sitter or do they have access to a reasonably equipped kitchen? Do they have a fridge or a deep freeze? What cooking methods do they use? How often do they use the frying pan or deep fryer? How often do they prepare foods from basic ingredients? Questions such as these may help you to understand the activities associated with how people are eating.

Retail sales

Rather than ask what people are consuming it may be easier to work out an average or overall pattern by asking what are they buying. Retailers need to keep good records of what they are selling and may be prepared to give you information. Sales at hospital staff restaurants or works canteens may be a simple way of detecting broadly based changes in eating habits. Chapter 14 gives more information on the advantages and disadvantages of using this sort of information.

Availability of food in local shops

The food choices people make depend not only on themselves but also on what is available for them to choose. It will help you to know what foods the local shops (or the shops which people regularly use) stock. What price compared with alternatives are the foods in which you are most interested? How visible are they in the shops? Are they tucked away on the top shelf in a corner, or are they at eye level in the busiest part of the shop? Are they promoted with posters and displays or is it left to the customer to seek them out? Promotions of healthier eating are more likely to succeed if you know the answers to questions like these.

Eating out

Eating out is becoming increasingly common. Questions therefore need to be asked about the restaurants and fast food places in your locality. What is on the menu and what is chosen most frequently? Are healthier choices available and are they identified on the menu? Is all the cooking heavy with butter and cream? Are salads and fresh fruits offered? What is the clientele of these establishments? Similar questions also need to be asked about the local works staff restaurants or canteens.

Background data

When collecting information from people you will want to know certain things about them in addition to what they are eating and what they think about food. This information will help you see if there are differences between groups. For example do men eat differently from women or the elderly differently from young people? Other people looking at your results will also want to know more about the people you were studying. At the very least you will want to know their age group, sex, ethnic group and area of residence.

In health surveys a great deal of attention has been paid to social class and interesting differences in disease frequency and lifestyle are found. The classification used by the Registrar General is shown in Box 2.3. This way of grouping people is based on their occupation (or sometimes for women their husband's occupation). Many other important things like educational level and income are thought to be associated with social class. However, there is a lot of dispute as to how helpful this social class grouping really is. Some of the other background data which might be useful for grouping and describing people and which you should also consider collecting are listed in Box 1.5.

Weight and other anthropometric measurements

Measurement of weight and height is needed in surveys intended to estimate the prevalence of obesity and the need for weight control. People may be asked to report their own weight and height but more accurate data will be obtained if the measurements are made by properly trained survey workers using properly calibrated instruments and standardised techniques. Other measurements such as waist and hip circumference and skinfold thickness add further useful information. However their measurement will add considerably to the time necessary for data collection and the survey staff must be trained in the use of standardised techniques. Ways of estimating body weight and adiposity data are shown in Box 2.4.

Physical examination and blood tests

When planning your study you may decide to collect information in additional ways to asking questions. Blood pressure is often included in health surveys but if this is done the blood pressure must be properly measured using standardised techniques. Some big surveys have included physical examination of the subjects but this takes a great deal of time and rarely yields worthwhile information on nutritional status.

A list of biochemical and haematological tests on blood samples which may be a useful addition to nutrition studies is given in Box 2.5. However, they are outside the scope of this book and if you want to find out more about them you

Box 2.4

Field estimates of adiposity and overweight

1 *Relative Weight*
   Weight as proportion of average 'desirable' weight for height
   Weight greater than 120% 'desirable'* weights is associated with
   appreciably increased risk

2 *Quetelet's Index (Body Mass Index – BMI)*
   Weight in kilogrammes divided by square of height in metres
   'Desirable'* BMI range 20-25kg/m^2
   BMI greater than 30 is associated with appreciably increased risk

3 *Waist: Hip ratio*
   Ratio of waist circumference to hip circumference
   'Desirable'* range less than 0.8 in women and less than 1.0 in men.
   This is a measure of central adiposity i.e. intra- and extra-abdominal fat
   which is thought to be the main source of cardiovascular risk from obesity

4 *Skinfold thickness*
   Measured with Harpenden or similar callipers usually at four sites (biceps,
   triceps, suprailiac, subscapular)
   These are a measure of subcutaneous adiposity

*N.B. 'Desirable' ranges need to be interpreted with caution. They are approximate
guides and apply to the generality of the population but are not appropriate for
everyone (e.g. many elite athletes do not fall within the 'desirable' range of BMI).

will have to look up more specialist books. Remember that if you are going to take blood samples it will not only add considerably to the cost of your study but also make it much more complicated to organise. People are also a good deal less likely to co-operate with your study if you ask them for a blood sample.

Mortality and morbidity

The main reason for our concern about what people are eating is the belief that this affects their health. So shouldn't we be collecting information about their health and illnesses? The most easily collected information about illness in a community are death statistics. Information on causes of death are routinely collected and published by HMSO in 'Causes of Death' which can be found in any large medical library. The Public Health Medicine department in your health district will also have information on the causes of death in the district.

Box 2.5

Blood tests of nutritional status

A   *Haematological*
Haemoglobin, Mean Corpuscular Haemoglobin Concentration (MCHC)
Mean Corpuscular Volume (MCV) Total White Cell Count
Serum Iron, Total Iron Binding Capacity (TIBC)
Serum Folate, Red Cell Folate, Serum B12

B   *Serum proteins*
Serum proteins, Albumin, Retinol Binding Protein (RBP)

C   *Blood lipids*
Cholesterol and lipid profiles

D   *Vitamin levels in plasma*
Ascorbic acid (and Leukocyte Ascorbic Acid)
Pyridoxine*
Retinol and Carotenes*
25-Hydroxycholecalciferol*
Vitamin E*

E   *Enzyme activation coefficients as measures of vitamin status*
Erythrocyte Glutathione Reductase Activation Coefficient (EGRAC for
riboflavin)*
Transkelotase Activation Coefficient (TKAC for thiamine)*
Red Cell Aspartate amino transferase (AATAC for pyridoxine)*

*Tests marked with a star are unlikely to be routinely available in district general
hospital laboratories and you will have to send samples to a laboratory specialising in
nutritional assessment or make other special arrangements.

Information on non-fatal illnesses (morbidity) is more difficult to come by.
Information on hospital admissions is collected through the Hospital Activity
Analysis (HAA) and regularly published by HMSO in the 'Hospital Inpatient
Enquiry' which will be found in all large medical libraries. The Public Health
Medicine department will also hold more information on admissions to the local
hospitals.

There is no generally available source of information on illness which does not
result in admission to hospital. A few general practices also act as 'spotter'
practices for the Royal College of General Practitioners and collect data on their

consultations. Discussion with the local Public Health Medicine department may reveal other useful local information such as outpatient surveys or surveys of general practice consultations. The regular publications from HMSO on morbidity and mortality are listed in Box 2.6.

Information on mortality and morbidity will be useful background to show how common nutrition related diseases are in your area. However, most diet related diseases take many, many years to develop. It is therefore very unlikely that death or disease rates would be measurably affected by health promotion activity in less than ten years. Furthermore the number of people in any health district who die prematurely of even common diseases is relatively small. In a typical district of 200,000 we would expect about a hundred people per year to die of heart disease before their 65th birthday.

With numbers of this size we have little chance of detecting the sort of changes which could realistically be achieved in the time scale of a year or two. The smallest difference between two years' figures which you could be reasonably sure of detecting (95% confidence limits) is about 40%. For these reasons morbidity and mortality are unlikely to be helpful for monitoring and evaluating healthier eating promotion activities except on a regional or national scale. Changes in death rates over time can be detected in national mortality statistics but it is extremely difficult to determine to what extent these are due to health promotion activity and to what extent due to other factors.

Deciding what information to collect

Be wary of broad intentions simply to collect information on nutritional beliefs, dietary health values, eating habits, food choices or nutrient intakes. Such a plan is unlikely to provide valid information which can be used to improve services or promote healthier eating or demonstrate the need for such activity.

In choosing what information to collect remember that the purpose of collecting it is to use it. Information about eating and the knowledge, attitudes and circumstances that affect eating may be used to check the need for new or different health promotion activity, to identify relevant activities and target populations, to find ways of improving existing activities or to decide whether old ones should be continued. At the end it must be possible to interpret the information gathered in a way that is relevant to the initial purpose.

The best way to start designing your study is by planning the sorts of questions that you need to answer in your report at the end and the conclusions that you hope to be able to make. Then select the items of information to collect and ways of collecting them that will enable you to establish or refute these conclusions. There is no point in collecting data to which the only possible reaction is 'so what?' or still worse data that cannot be interpreted at all.

Box 2.6

Some sources of background statistical information

A large range of health and statistical data is produced by the OPCS (Office of Population Census and Surveys) for the Government and published by HMSO, including the following:

1   Data on deaths (Mortality)
There are 5 series published annually on different aspects of mortality data in England and Wales.

Series DH1. Review of deaths
        DH2. Cause of death
        DH5. Deaths by Area (Tables are on microfiche)

DH1 and DH2 give overviews of the national picture. Series DH5 will probably be most relevant to district studies: it shows deaths broken down by diagnostic group of registered cause of death and age sex group for each Health District and Local Authority area.

2   Hospital Inpatient Data
Series MB4 Hospital Inpatient Enquiry (H.I.P.E.) – Tables are on microfiche

This is published annually and shows data on number of discharges, discharge rate and length of stay from Hospitals in England and Wales broken down by diagnostic group and age/sex group for each Health District.

3   Cancer statistics
Series MB1 Cancer statistics

This is published annually and gives cancer registrations and other cancer data for England and Wales. It is based on reports from the Cancer Registries.

4   Population statistics
The main source of population statistics is the census reports published every 10 years. This gives a large amount of data on local populations at the time of the census. As one gets further away from the census year the data become progressively less accurate.

Continued overleaf

29

Box 2.6 (Continued)

5 *Series VS Key and Population statistics*
This is published annually and gives various updates and projections
(estimated changes in population) for areas and districts.

6 *Data on Scotland and Northern Ireland*
The data sources listed above refer to England and Wales. Corresponding data
for Scotland and Ireland can be found in:
      Annual Report of the Registrar General for Scotland
and
      Northern Ireland Report

7 *Decennial supplements*
These reports are published irregularly and cover a range of topics linking
death and other data to census data. The following reports are of particular
relevance:

Life tables   – Showing life expectancy

Occupational mortality   – Differences in mortality between occupational
                                   groups and differences between social classes

8 *Data from General Practice*
There is no regular national report on morbidity seen in general practice but
see the reports of the National Morbidity Surveys.

RCGP and OPCS (1979). Morbidity Statistics from General Practice 1971-72.
2nd National Morbidity Survey. Studies on medical and population subjects
No. 36.

RCGP and OPCS (1986). Morbidity Statistics from General Practice. 3rd
National Study. Series MB5 No. 1.

9 *General Household Survey*
This is an annual survey covering many aspects of lifestyle (different aspects
are covered in different years) including smoking, drinking, taking of
medication, and days of illness and disability. Much of this data is broken
down to the regional level (but not to Health District level).

10 *National Food Survey*
This is described in more detail in Box 12.8.

Information for evaluation studies

Evaluation studies are concerned with the questions:
   Have things changed?
   Have your health promotion activities influenced that change?
   Have the health promotion objectives been achieved?
   Why was the activity successful or unsuccessful?

The information which must be collected for an evaluation study will be in part specified by the health promotion objectives. However, you may also need to collect information on subjects not mentioned in the objectives if you want to understand why the objectives were or were not achieved. For example, if your health promotion objective was to change knowledge or eating behaviour then information on awareness of your activities, credibility of your materials and beliefs and values favourable or antagonistic to your efforts may all help evaluation. There is more discussion on the choice of variables for evaluation studies in the section on study design in Chapter 4.

And finally

This chapter has given a very long list of types of information you might want to collect. You will have to pick out just a few. Remember the reason for collecting information is to use it. So if you can't think why you want it, don't collect it.

Box 2.7

Questionnaire on food beliefs

A great number of things have been suggested as being wrong with the way people eat today. This page contains a long list of them. Please will you say whether you agree or disagree with these statements.

Please ring one response
for each statement

A Definitely agree
B Probably agree
C Neither agree nor disagree
D Probably disagree
E Definitely disagree

People in UK today are not eating enough organic food	A B C D E
People in UK today are not eating enough starch	A B C D E
People in UK today are not eating enough dietary fibre	A B C D E
People in UK today are not eating enough sugar	A B C D E
People in UK today are not eating enough fat	A B C D E
People in UK today are not eating enough vitamins	A B C D E
People in UK today are not eating enough minerals	A B C D E
People in UK today are not eating enough bread	A B C D E
People in UK today are not eating enough potatoes	A B C D E
People in UK today are not eating enough fresh fuit	A B C D E
People in UK today are not eating enough meat and meat products	A B C D E
People in UK today are not eating enough fish and sea foods	A B C D E
People in UK today don't get enough food to eat	A B C D E
We need better food labelling in UK today	A B C D E

Continued opposite

Box 2.7 (Continued)

Food is too expensive for people to afford in UK today   A   B   C   D   E

Irradiated food should not be allowed to be sold   A   B   C   D   E

Eggs sold in UK are not safe to eat   A   B   C   D   E

Most vegetables sold in UK contain dangerous amounts
    of pesticide   A   B   C   D   E

People in UK today are eating too many additives   A   B   C   D   E

People in UK today are eating too much salt   A   B   C   D   E

People in UK today are eating too much starch   A   B   C   D   E

People in UK today are eating too much sugar   A   B   C   D   E

People in UK today are eating too much fat   A   B   C   D   E

People in UK today are drinking too much alcohol   A   B   C   D   E

People in UK today are eating too much dietary fibre   A   B   C   D   E

People in UK today are eating too many foods
    with E numbers   A   B   C   D   E

People in UK today are eating too many sweets   A   B   C   D   E

People in UK today are eating too much fresh fruit   A   B   C   D   E

People in UK today are eating too many dairy products   A   B   C   D   E

People in UK today are eating too much meat and
    meat products   A   B   C   D   E

People in UK today are eating too much bread   A   B   C   D   E

People in UK today are eating too much processed food   A   B   C   D   E

People in UK today are eating too much fattening food   A   B   C   D   E

Continued overleaf

Further reading

Setting agendas

French J. and Adams L. (1986). 'Theories of health education.'
Health Education Journal 45, 71-74.

Tones K. (1987). Health education, PSE and the question of voluntarism.
Journal of Institute of Health Education 25, 41-52.

Social class gradients health

Townsend P. and Davidson N. (1988). 'Inequalities in Health.'
The Black Report (1980) and The Health Divide – Whitehead M. Publ. Penguin.

The effect of health promotion on mortality

Goldman L. and Cook E. F. (1984). 'The decline in ischaemic heart disease
mortality rates: An analysis of the effect of medical interventions and
changes in lifestyle.'
Annals of Internal Medicine 101, 825-826

Anthropometric measures

Weiner J. S. and Lowrie S. A. (1969). *Human Biology. A guide to field methods* IBP Handbook No. 9. Publ. Blackwell Scientific, Oxford.

Biochemical assessment of nutritional status

Sauberlich H. E., Dowdy R. P. and Skala J. H. (1974). *Laboratory tests for the assessment of nutritional status*. CRC Press, Florida.

Thurnham D. (1985). 'Biochemical assessment of nutritional status.' In Kemm J. R. (Ed.) *Vitamin Deficiency in the Elderly*. Publ. Blackwell Scientific, Oxford.

Health consequences of obesity

Working Party of the Royal College of Physicians (1983). 'Obesity.' *Journal of Royal College of Physicians of London* 17, 5-65.

3 · Planning the study – Writing the protocol

Summary

This first step in any study should be writing down what you want to do and how you propose to do it. This written plan of action is called a protocol.

This chapter describes the pieces of information which should be included in a protocol.

What is a protocol?

A protocol is a written plan of investigation. It is rather like the plans for building a house. It tells you what the finished product will look like, the different parts that make up the final product, the order in which things are to be done and the resources which are needed to do the job. The things which ought to be in a protocol are shown in Box 3.1.

Before you begin – preliminary enquiries

Before you try to design any study or write any protocol, you should get a 'feel' for the problem you are considering tackling. There is nothing like exploratory enquiries for informing study design in a new area. The purpose of these enquiries is to clarify the broad issues. They will also ensure that when you come to report your results you know why they are important and can make suggestions as to what ought to be done about them.

Take just an hour or two for a few conversations with ordinary people who are unaware of your intended investigation. Choose one or two people of the type that you are thinking about studying. Ask them about what they actually do. Direct the conversation to activities like eating, food preparation and shopping but don't focus exclusively on your interest – get a fair context. Try to find out something about why the person does what they do. If possible avoid directly asking why they do things but find this out indirectly by asking what they would do in slightly different circumstances. For example, would they ever take the skin off chicken before cooking, and why do they do this or not do it? What type(s) of cheese do they eat and what are the attractions in each?

This qualitative interviewing does not have to be 'deep' or 'psychological'. You are only trying to expose yourself to the more obvious factors in the food choices. It is important that the conversation is not prejudicial or directive. Above all don't let your views on what is healthy eating creep into the interview as this will bias your findings.

It is all too easy to get stuck in the thinking, talking and reading. Ideas change so often and life is so complicated that there is a danger that you never feel ready to start collecting data. Collecting a little information very informally will help you get started with the actual design of the study.

Why write a protocol?

The main reason for writing a protocol is that it forces you to plan your study properly. This planning should cover the whole process from preliminary enquiries right through to final completion and production of an effective report. It helps you to be clear as to what you are trying to achieve and to check that you are using the methods and collecting the sort of data that will enable you to achieve your objective.

It should help you anticipate the difficulties that you are likely to encounter in doing the study and to identify the time, manpower and equipment that you will need. Time spent writing the protocol will reduce the chances of starting a study that cannot be completed or could not possibly achieve its aims.

A second use of the protocol comes if you have to seek permission from your manager for the study or to apply for funds or other resources for your study. Management and funding agencies will want to be persuaded that you have sensible questions and a plan of study that will enable you to answer those questions. They will also want you to explain how you propose to spend their money on staff, equipment etc., and why these are needed for the study. A well written protocol is an essential part of any grant application.

Where to begin writing the protocol

This chapter is constructed as though writing a protocol were a straightforward operation beginning with a statement of aims and proceeding logically through setting objectives to deciding what data to collect and methods of collecting them and ending with the resources required. Real life is not like that. In practice when you get to methods or resources you are likely to find that you cannot do what you originally intended. Then you have to go back and adjust your aims to match your resources. You will probably have to go through this cycle several times before you arrive at a protocol which is a compromise between what you first wanted to do and what you can realistically do with the resources at your disposal. You will also find that this process of reviewing and adjusting your protocol sharpens your original ideas and may well make your study more informative and useful.

Box 3.1

What is in a protocol?

Title of study

What is the study for?
Aims and objectives
Type of study – analytic or descriptive
Specific hypotheses to be tested (in analytic studies)

Background
Literature survey
Information on the local situation

Target population
Sampling frame – method of sampling – size of sample

Data collection
Variables to be measured
Methods of measuring variables

Approach for analysing results
Outline tables
Statistical treatment of results
How hypotheses will be tested

Use of results
In what form will they be reported?
Who will be informed of results?

Resources and costs
Personnel – supervision, field workers, coding, data entry, analysis, report
    writing etc.
Consumables – printing, postage, telephones, travel, etc.
Computing capacity

Timetable
Pilot studies
Main study

Is consent of ethical committee or other bodies required?

Pilot study

Your first protocol should include at least one pilot study. Even if you are applying a study design that has been worked out elsewhere in your district, the methods will still need to be tested in the situation in which you propose to use them.

If you are designing a study virtually from scratch, there will be several things which you need to find out before you can finalise your plan for the main study. Will your questionnaires gather the required information? How many interviews can a field worker complete in a day? What response rate can you expect? These questions can only be answered by trying out your initial ideas in a small pilot study. You can then use the information gathered in the pilot study to make further improvements to the protocol for the main study.

Sometimes the pilot study will show that there is a fundamental problem in your protocol and lead you to change your plans radically. It may show that you need to change your methods or even your aims and objectives. One of the reasons for doing pilot studies is to find out problems before you waste a lot of time, effort and money on an unworkable study.

Getting help

When you try to write a protocol you may well decide that you need advice from some of the people listed in Box 3.2. The time to seek help is at the planning stage before the study. There is usually nothing anyone can do to rescue the situation when presented with a pile of results from a badly designed study.

Box 3.2

People whose advice might be helpful for research on healthy eating

Statistician
Epidemiologist
Clinical or applied social psychologist
Nutritional anthropologist or sociologist
Market researcher
Health educationalist
Dietician
Anyone with expertise relevant to the topic of the study.

A statistician can help in all sorts of ways. They will be able to advise not just on sample size and methods of data analysis but on all aspects of formal design of the study.

Aims

The first thing to decide is what are you trying to do in general terms. Your aim might be something like 'to find out about consumption of dietary fibre in Central Birmingham Health District' or 'to find out whether there was any change in staff attitudes following your hospital's healthy eating campaign'. If you have been asked to do the study by someone else then you will need to clarify with them exactly what they wish the study to achieve.

Setting objectives

The aims tell us the broad area with which the study will be concerned but they do not say precisely what questions are to be answered. This is the purpose of the next step, setting the objectives. These objectives will be narrower than the general aim but will say exactly what the study is going to do.

For the study whose aim was to find out about dietary fibre consumption the objectives might be 'to describe the range of individuals' frequency of consumption of different types of bread, vegetables and fruit' and 'to find if frequency of consumption of these foods differs between age and sex groups'. For the study of change following the hospital's healthy eating campaign the objectives might be 'to compare the value that nursing and medical staff attach to healthier eating before and immediately after the campaign'.

Testing hypotheses

In many studies we will be looking for differences between groups, for changes over time or for both. The general approach used to test whether there really is a change or a difference is called testing the 'null hypothesis'. This is explained further in Box 3.3.

Type of study

Studies may be descriptive or analytical. Descriptive studies simply describe the characteristics of a group and answer questions like 'what proportion of residents in this district drink skimmed or semi-skimmed milk?' or 'What proportion of hospital staff remember seeing the District's healthy eating posters?'.

41

Box 3.3

Testing the null hypothesis

'Testing the null hypothesis' involves calculating how likely we would be to get results like the ones we have obtained if there really were no difference.

If it appears that we are very unlikely to have obtained our results if there really were no difference then we say that the null hypothesis has been rejected and we conclude that there probably is a real difference.

Examples of null hypotheses might be:
'There is no difference between the frequency of consumption of wholemeal bread by men aged 20 to 39 and by men aged 40 to 59'.
'There is no difference in the knowledge score of nurses in the hospital before and after the healthy eating campaign'.
'There is no difference in the proportion of people who use low fat spreads in this district and the proportion nationally'.

These null hypotheses need to be stated at the protocol writing stage.

If the null hypothesis is not rejected
If the null hypothesis is not rejected we cannot conclude that there is no difference. All that can be said is that our method did not detect any difference.

Analytical studies look for differences between groups or changes over time. Analytical studies answer questions like 'Is the percent energy derived from fat greater in white men than in Asian men?' or 'Is the knowledge of dietary risk factors for coronary heart disease increased after the Look After Your Heart Campaign?' or 'Are people who know dietary risk factors for coronary heart disease more likely to choose low fat foods than people who do not know them?'. Analytical studies tend to be more difficult to design than descriptive studies but are often much more useful. Most studies are a mixture of descriptive and analytical.

Monitoring and evaluation studies are a special type of analytic study and their design raises particular problems which are discussed in the next chapter.

Background literature

An important part of planning your study is the literature search. Before you go further than setting a general aim you need to find out what other people have written about the subject. Almost certainly someone has attempted a similar study before and their findings can guide you as to what you might expect to find, what variables you should be studying and what methods you could use.

Other people's work may be reported in one of the scientific journals or in an unpublished report produced for their colleagues. You can usually find where the original reports were published by looking in books or review articles in journals. When you have located the original reports you should check whether there have been more recent follow-up studies. Other people interested in the subject of your study will probably be able to tell you where you can find reports of interesting surveys. Once you have found one or two reports, you can probably find more by looking up the references to earlier reports given in the reports that you have found. You could also write to the authors of the most

---

Box 3.4

Special aids for literature searches

1 *The Index Medicus*
   The Index Medicus is an index to virtually all papers published in medical journals. Each month a volume the size of a large telephone directory is published showing the most recent additions to the index under topic areas. Other indexes are also published.

2 *Computer searches*
   Computer searches for papers have also become widely available and they will enable you to find large numbers of papers on any subject.

3 *Citation indexes*
   Citation indexes (particularly I.S.I.) are indexes which show which recently published papers have cited (made reference to) earlier publications. If you know one or two key papers published a few years ago, then looking up the recent papers which have cited them can be a very efficient way of finding more recent work on the same subject.

A word of caution
There are two problems with using the Index Medicus or similar indexes or computerised searches. First they produce a very large number of papers including several that may be irrelevant or for some other reason not worth reading. Second they rely on the original indexing and so may miss some important papers. Unless you know the subject well the Index Medicus or a computerised search will probably not be the best place to start your search.

---

relevant reports to ask if they can tell you of any more recent studies on the topic.

When choosing the methods of data collection you will need to see what methods other people have used. You may choose to use a method developed by someone else and you will then need to see exactly how they collected their data and what evidence they present that their method works. If you decide to develop your own method, you will need to justify this decision by showing that the methods used by others did not work or are not suitable for your purposes.

A visit to the nearest medical or university library is worthwhile. If you explain what you are looking for, the librarian can tell you how to find the relevant papers. University and polytechnic libraries have various aids to finding papers on any subject (see Box 3.4). Your librarian should be able to advise you on the use of these aids.

The local situation

The local situation will also be an important influence on the planning of your study. Has anyone in your organisation compiled any local data on the subject? Have any surveys been done before? Are there any reasons for thinking your district is different from the national situation? If for example you wanted to study iron intakes then it would be helpful to know how many cases of iron deficiency anaemia had been diagnosed in the district. Box 3.5 gives an example of the local information which might be useful when planning a survey of dietary risk factors for ischaemic heart disease in a district.

Target population and sampling

Defining the population to be studied and how they are to be sampled is a crucial part of survey design and must be included in the protocol. This subject is fully discussed in Chapter 7.

Variables to be measured and method of measurement

A long list of variables in which you might be interested was given in Chapter 2 and methods for measuring different sorts of variables are described in Chapters 9 to 13.

Methods of analysis

A recurrent theme of this book is that the only reason for collecting data is to use them. It follows that you should have a clear idea what you are going to do with your findings when you have collected them. It is often useful to draw up

Box 3.5

Local background information for survey of dietary risk factors for Ischaemic Heart Disease (IHD)

Example of Central Birmingham Health District

Age specific death rates for IHD in 1986 (per 1000)

Age	35-44	45-54	55-64	65-74	75-84
Male	0.4	2.9	8.1	18.1	27.2
Female	0.1	0.7	1.6	6.4	15.7

Age standarised mortality ratio (25-74) with 95% confidence limits for IHD in different wards (1983-86)

	Male	Female
Quinton	98 (81-118)	81 (58-110)
Harborne	81 (65-99)	92 (69-120)
Edgbaston	105 (85-128)	105 (76-141)
Nechells	110 (91-132)	100 (71-136)
Sparkbrook	122 (101-146)	132 (94-178)
Sparkhill	114 (93-138)	94 (64-133)
Fox Hollies	102 (85-122)	107 (81-138)
National	100	100

Consumption of various foodstuffs

(No local data available – West Midlands data from National Food Survey 1985)

	West Midlands	National	
Milk and cream	4.1	4.1	pt/wk
Cheese	4.4	3.9	oz/wk
Meat and meat products	37.2	36.8	oz/wk
Fats and oils	10.2	10.3	oz/wk

Nutrient intake

(No local data available – West Midlands data from National Food Survey 1985)

	West Midlands	National	
Energy	2110	2020	kcal/day
Fat	97	96	g/day
Saturated fatty acids	41.0	40.6	g/day
Monounsaturated fatty acids	35.4	34.7	g/day
Polyunsaturated fatty acids	13.5	13.1	g/day
% Energy from fat	37.9	39.1	%

dummy tables showing how you propose to look at your results when you have got them. An example of this is given in Box 3.6. You must be clear what conclusions you hope to draw from these tables and how these conclusions will help you plan health promotion activities or other services.

When drawing up dummy tables you should check how many observations there will probably be in each cell of the table or each subgroup. You can then see whether you are likely to have sufficient numbers to allow comparisons between groups.

You should also decide whether you are going to process your results with pen, paper and hand calculator (which is very adequate for simple surveys) or whether you are going to use a computer.

Resources – time

It is infuriating when you are half-way through a study to find that you cannot finish it because you haven't enough time. Before you start you need to identify all the jobs that have to be done, how long they will take to do and who will do them.

If the study involves interviewing people, remember that you have to allow time for people to talk about things other than the interview (friendly time) and time for travel. If other people are helping you with the survey, you must allow time for training and then time for liaison and administrative work. The time requirements for a dietary survey are further discussed in Chapter 12. You will have to allow time for checking that report forms have been properly completed and coded. If you are using a computer time is needed to enter the data onto the computer and for checking for mistakes once they have been entered. A lot of time will be needed for analysis of the results and writing up the report. When writing the protocol you should check that you have made adequate arrangements for all these tasks. For some tasks you may not know how much time is required and therefore need to do small pilot studies to find out how long it will take you to do the task.

Other resources

In addition to time, most surveys use other resources. Forms have to be printed or copied. If people are to be visited at home, travel costs may be considerable. If it is a postal questionnaire then there will be postage costs. All these requirements should be identified before you start and you should know how you are going to cover them. If you are planning to lose them by putting them in the general overheads of your job, then you should check that no one is going to object to this later.

Box 3.6

Examples of dummy tables

Question – Does bread consumption differ between age groups?
Separate table for males and females

Reported number of slices eaten per day

Age	0-2	3-4	5-6	7-8	8+
20-44					
45-64					
65+					

Reported type of bread usually eaten

Age	White	Wholemeal	Other Brown	Mixture
20-44				
45-64				
65+				

Question – Does bread consumption differ between wards?
Similar tables as above with wards instead of ages.

Question – Do the ward populations have different age structures?

	Age group		
	20-44	45-64	65+
Ward 1			
Ward 2			
Ward 3			
Ward 4			
Etc.			

Question – Could the difference in wards be due to their different population age structures?
The simplest approach is to draw up for each ward separate tables as above for number of slices and usual type of bread by age group. Will this give very small numbers in each table? If so you need either to find a more powerful way of analysing your data or to increase the sample size.

These sorts of problem should be identified and discussed with a statistician before you start to collect the data.

Use of computers

If you are going to use a computer then you will need to check that it has the software to do the things that you want. Remember you have to allow time and make arrangements for both data entry and performing the analysis.

If you are going to do the computing yourself you need to check that the machine will be available for you to work on it. You can probably use one of the programme packages available for personal computers (such as SPSSPC or Minitab). These packages will do most of the tabulations and statistical calculations that you require. You will want to try out the package that you intend to use and check that it provides the outputs that you want.

If you are expecting someone else to do the computing, you need to agree with them what computing is to be done on your data. You must be sure that they have left enough time in their work schedules for the job. Jobs which are going to be done 'when someone has a spare moment' usually take a very long time to get done.

It cannot be too strongly emphasised that there is no point whatever in collecting any data unless it can be coded, summarised, analysed, interpreted and written up in a report within a few months.

Timetable

When you know what you want to do and what resources you have to do it with you can plan the timetable for the study. If the results are wanted for a particular deadline you can check that you will be able to produce on time.

This timetable will help you see if the study is going as you intended and to take early remedial action if you encounter difficulties. An example of a study timetable is shown in Box 3.7.

Permissions and co-operation

Many Health Districts like all research proposals to be considered by the Medical Ethical Committee. You need to consider whether your study will need ethical permission.

You may also need permission from other people. If you are going to question hospital employees then the Unit General Manager and probably the Union representative may need to be approached. If you want to study patients in hospital you will probably need to obtain the permission of their Consultants. If you want to look at school children's eating pattern in schools you will need the

Box 3.7

Example of study timetable

Outline of study

Aim:	To assess the adequacy of diet of mothers of single parent families in an urban area.
Method:	Use of food frequency and habits questionnaire (questionnaire already developed and validated) to be completed at interview in subject's home.
Study population:	All such mothers on list of one General Practitioner (expected number 30).
Personnel:	Yourself full time for 4 months; Assistance with data entry.
Data analysis:	To be done on personal computer using statistical package.

Timetable

Preparation before fieldwork
1. Do literature search, collect background data.
   Plan study, write protocol.   3 weeks
2. Visit GP, explain project to primary care team.
   Identify list of mothers.   1 week
3. Check questionnaire suitable for target group.
   Assess time needed for each interview.   1 week

Fieldwork
4. Send letters to subjects to arrange interview.   1 week
5. Do interviews.
   Half hour interview, half hour social time. One hour travel.
   Half hour office work check and code questionnaire,
   30 interviews allowing for missed appointments etc.   4 weeks

Continued overleaf

Box 3.7 (Continued)

After fieldwork – Analysis and report writing

6   Data entry 15 minutes per form.
    One and a half days work for data entry assistant.   —

7   Preliminary analysis using package.
    Inspection of preliminary results.   1 week

8   Outline drafting of report.
    Further analysis based on preliminary findings.
    Further literature search.   2 weeks

9   Finalise report.   1 week

10 Disseminate results – seminar to interested groups etc.   3 weeks

Total

Preparation before fieldwork	5 weeks
Fieldwork	5 weeks
After fieldwork analysis and report writing	7 weeks

Note these timings assume that:

1   You will spend most of your time on the project.

2   You don't need to pilot and develop the questionnaire but have one ready to use.

3   The G.P. has already agreed in principle to co-operate with the study.

permission of the Local Education Authority and then the head teachers (see Chapter 15).

You will also need good co-operation from the operational staff (nurses, health visitors, teachers, catering staff etc). They will be helping you to get your interviews, make your observations or get your questionnaires completed and collected. You must negotiate with them about the way in which you will collect your data and how your work will fit in with their duties.

4 · Study design for monitoring and evaluation

Summary

Good study design is essential to provide data that can be interpreted and meet the objectives of the study. Confounding variables are variables which interfere with the effect of the factor that we are trying to study. Monitoring studies investigate change over time. Evaluation studies examine the effect of health promotion activity and seek to establish the cause of any change observed.

Several study designs may be used to study cause but all rely on comparison of groups which receive the intervention (health promotion activity) with control groups. The features of the different designs are described and discussed.

What is study design?

Information should always be collected for some purpose such as helping you plan more effective health promotion campaigns or assessing the effectiveness of completed or continuing activities. If information is to be useful in this way the study in which it is collected must be properly designed. Badly designed studies yield data which cannot be used to answer the questions with which the study was concerned or worse still cannot be interpreted at all.

Study design covers all aspects of what information is collected and how it is collected. Choosing which variables to study (Chapter 2), devising valid methods of measurement (Chapter 5) and planning appropriate samples of adequate size (Chapter 7) are all part of study design.

Design back from the end

Study design begins with deciding what questions we intend to answer when the study is completed. We must then identify what information could be interpreted in a way that would answer the initial questions and would make it possible to rule out alternative interpretations. So the best way to design a study is to work backwards from the subjects on which we wish to make conclusions through the information needed to reach those conclusions to plans for gathering that information.

Confounding

Nearly all analytic studies attempt to examine the effect of some factor such as

51

gender, age, employment status, time or health promotion activity on some other variables. Unfortunately there are nearly always other interfering factors which also affect the variables in which we are interested. These other factors are called confounding variables (or less politely 'confounded nuisances'!). If confounding variables are forgotten or neglected you will end up with data that cannot be interpreted.

For example, suppose you wished to know if men and women differed in their knowledge of risk factors for heart disease. You have measured this knowledge in a group of men and a group of women and found that the women's knowledge was greater. However you also found that the women were appreciably younger than the men. Age is then a confounding variable and you cannot be sure (without more information) whether being female or being younger or both is associated with greater knowledge of the risk factors.

In monitoring studies the factor whose effect we are trying to study is time, while in evaluation studies the factor of interest is health promotion activity. The purpose of study design is to enable us to distinguish the effect of these variables from that of possible confounding variables.

Design of monitoring studies – have things changed over time?

Monitoring is concerned with the question whether things such as knowledge and beliefs about food and health, foods eaten, availability of foods and so on have changed over time. The basic study design involves making two or more measurements of the variable of interest and comparing the results. The essential requirement is to obtain comparable measurements so that the effect of time can be distinguished from that of other confounding variables.

Suppose you want to know whether the proportion of your district population who drink skimmed milk is changing. Six months ago you took a sample of 200 people and asked them about what type of milk they used and you have just repeated the exercise with a new sample of 200 people. You find that the proportion who report drinking skimmed milk is 15% greater in the second sample than in the one taken six months ago. Does this mean that the proportion drinking skimmed milk has increased or could the difference in milk consumption be due to the effect of some confounding variable? In fact the two samples turn out to be not strictly comparable and you note that the second sample differs from the first in various ways. The proportion of women is higher, the proportion in non-manual jobs is higher and the average age is lower. All of these factors could be associated with a higher proportion of skimmed milk drinkers. In this case, without more information you cannot be sure that the proportion of milk drinkers in the population has changed.

You may decide to try and avoid the difficulty of obtaining comparable samples by seeking information from the same people on more than one occasion. For example, in the study of skimmed milk consumption you might have returned to the same people whom you asked first time to find out about their milk drinking six months later. However if you found that more of them now report drinking skimmed milk you still could not be sure that this is generally true of the population in your district. Maybe the process of answering our questions about milk consumption first time round has made some of them think and stimulated them to change the type of milk they drink. It could also be that some people are now more or less willing to report their milk drinking habits accurately (a change in social acceptability bias – see Chapter 12 page xx). For all of these reasons a change in the proportion of our sample who report drinking skimmed milk is not necessarily a reliable indicator that things have changed in the population. Appropriate design is needed so that we can distinguish the effect of time from that of other confounding variables.

Usually the variable which we want to measure is constantly changing so that two measurements at different points of time do not give us an adequate picture of what is happening. Often the question we want to ask is not whether something is changing but whether it is changing faster or slower than before. (In other words has the rate of change altered?) Plotting repeated measurements over time is a good way of showing trends (see Figure 4.1).

Once again if you are contemplating a study to find out whether something is changing over time you will find it very helpful to discuss its design with a statistician.

Figure 4.1   Trends in consumption of different foods

Source: National Food Survey

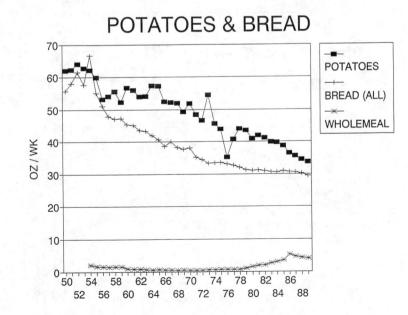

POTATOES & BREAD

Figure 4.1 (continued)

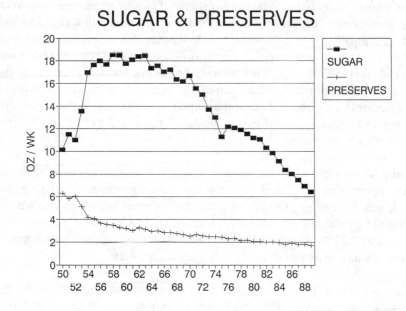

SUGAR & PRESERVES

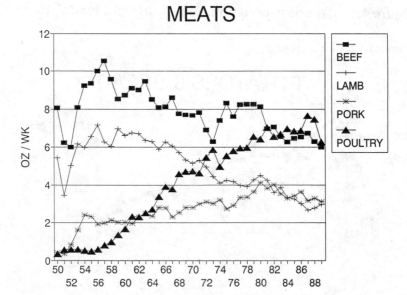

MEATS

Design for evaluation

Evaluation studies ask not only whether things have changed but also whether our health promotion activity has influenced that change. This helps sort out whether service activities are of some real value. The different types of evaluation were described in Chapter 1. Evaluation studies have to be designed so that the effect of health promotion activity can be distinguished from that of other confounding variables.

Design of evaluation studies in health promotion is difficult because there are usually a very large number of confounding variables to be considered. For example, we might wish to examine the effect of a campaign encouraging men not to drink more than 21 units of alcohol per week. However our campaign coincided with a strike at the brewery, an increase in the price of beer, a breathalyser campaign by the local police and a national advertising campaign by the Health Education Authority, all of which might be expected to depress consumption. It also coincided with a spell of hot weather and an advertising campaign by the brewers which might be expected to increase consumption. All of these things could be confounding variables. At the end of our campaign we would not know whether any observed change in alcohol consumption was due to our activity or to the other things (confounding variables) which happened at the same time. The study designs for investigating cause are described later in this chapter.

Interaction with national trends

Local health promotion activity is frequently confounded by national trends. Suppose you run a local programme to promote consumption of skimmed milk or wholemeal bread and consumption of these products rises during the programme. It is possible that this was an effect of the programme but a very widespread set of other influences could have produced the increase in consumption. The local promotion activity may have coincided with a national trend. The promotion activity may or may not have strengthened the trend locally but in these circumstances it is very difficult (and therefore expensive) to show whether the local activity has had any effect.

Comparison data may be hard to come by but some useful sources do exist. The National Food Survey (see Box 12.8), for example, may enable you to predict trends for consumption of different foods in your district on the basis that it will be expected to follow national trends.

Even if there is little chance of being able to tell whether your local health promotion activity has influenced trends there may still be good reasons to collect the data on consumption (and even to strengthen the design so that it could show the local effect). Publicly collecting the data may be a good way for the Health Service to show that it is interested, approves of the trend and wishes to encourage it. However do not pretend to yourself that this exercise will measure the effectiveness of District Food Policy.

Interaction with other local activities

Another common problem in interpreting evaluation studies is that the health promotion activity coincided with other local efforts. Indeed, a good food policy should include encouragement of efforts by other organisations, such as high street shops and eating places, pubs and clubs. Where several activities are taking place at the same time affecting the same people it is usually difficult or impossible to portion out which activity (health service or commercial) was responsible for which changes.

Causal inference

All study designs to investigate cause rely on comparision of those who have received the health promotion activity and those who have not. Comparison of the two groups allows the effects of the health promotion activity to be distinguished from effects of confounding variables. In studies of this type the thing whose effect is being investigated is usually called the 'intervention' so in this section we will refer to health promotion activities as the 'intervention'.

The designs fall into two groups. In experimental designs the investigator decides who shall receive the health promotion activity and who will not. In 'natural experiments' two pre-existing groups are compared and the investigator does not determine who shall receive the health promotion activity. The different designs available (Table 4.1) will now be described.

Table 4.1   Study designs for causal inference

Experimental
   Randomised controlled study
   Non-random comparison study
   Lagged comparisons between groups
Natural experiments
   Comparisons of selected groups within populations
   Predicted and non-predicted change (Multiple Baseline Studies)
   Comparison of different methods
Studies without comparison groups
   Trend analysis
   Before and after comparison

Randomised controlled studies

Theoretically the clearest way to find out whether an activity such as distributing leaflets or organising meetings is the cause of a change is to take two groups (samples). One group is subject to the health promotion activity and is called the intervention group. The other group is not subject to the activity and is called the control group. One then compares the two groups before and after the intervention period. The control group should be comparable with the intervention group in all respects except that it does not receive the activity. If before the intervention the two groups do not differ but after the intervention they do differ then we have very strong grounds for concluding that our intervention was the cause of the difference.

One key feature of this design is random allocation of people to intervention or control group. Every individual in the study has the same chance of being allocated to a particular group. This excludes potential biases. Random allocation is equivalent to random sampling and its theory and ways of doing it are described in Chapter 6.

If the intervention and control groups are formed by random allocation the variety of characteristics in each group should be similar and the only difference between them should be the intervention. However random allocation can still produce groups that differ by chance in some respects. This is especially true when group sizes are small. The comparability of groups should be checked for measurable characteristics such as age and especially for any characteristic that could produce an effect similar to that of the intervention. For example, if one were studying the effect of a leaflet distribution on nutritional knowledge, it would be important to check that things like educational level and newspaper readership were similar in the two groups.

Sometimes the subjects are matched (for age, sex, etc.) in pairs before random allocation and when the first member of a pair is allocated to one group the second member of that pair is allocated to the other group. This retains the freedom from bias but may give better comparability of groups.

Drop-outs and contamination

Even if you start with comparable groups, drop-out can cause problems. People can differ in their involvement in the activities being compared. If these people are not available for measurement at the end of the study period, the comparability of the groups will have been spoilt and an unknown bias will have been introduced. On the other hand dropping out is in itself a significant event and any health promotion activity which has a high drop-out rate needs to be reconsidered.

With long running programmes there is likely to be appreciable 'contamination' between groups so that the control group actually receive some of the activities intended only for the intervention group. This reduces the difference between the groups. An example of the problems caused by contamination was the Multiple Risk Factor Intervention Trial (MRFIT). This was a large American study with random allocation in which the intervention group were intended to receive among other things advice on healthier eating (cholesterol lowering diets). However the differences were less than expected and it was clear that the control group had also made considerable changes in their eating

Often random allocation just is not possible. For example, if running a local radio campaign it would be impossible to limit hearing the broadcast just to people in an intervention group. For events requiring appreciable participation, the subjects must be asked for informed consent to be randomly allocated and many will not agree to this.

Though attractive in theory randomised control designs are very rarely possible in practice.

Non-random comparison group studies

When it is not possible to obtain a randomly allocated control group another group which has not received the intervention may be taken as a comparison group. When there is a healthy eating programme in one district, another district in which there is no such programme may be taken for comparison. On a smaller scale, if a health promotion activity is targeted at one city ward or one school or one hospital, another ward, school or hospital may be taken as comparison group.

The problems with this design are first that no two health districts, city wards, schools or hospitals have identical populations. So one can never be absolutely sure that the two are really comparable or that any difference observed was due to the health promotion activity rather than to pre-existing differences between the comparison groups. In these circumstances it is very important to measure possible confounding variables such as age, family size, ethnicity and occupational status.

The second problem is that contamination is likely to occur and especially when the two groups are close to each other (e.g. two wards in the same city). The risk of contamination between groups may be reduced by wider geographical separation but this is likely to be at the expense of having groups that are less comparable.

Lagged comparison design

Studies of comparable Districts which begin comparable activities at different times allow us to distinguish the effects of an intervention from the effects of confounding variables. If the delay is long enough for the effect in the first District to be completed, then the later District provides an ordinary control. However, useful comparison is still possible if the activity starts in the second District while it is still continuing in the first District. Effects of national trends and events should occur at the same time in the two districts. On the other hand the growth in size and persistence over time of the effect of the intervention should occur in the second district later than in the first. The time interval between the effects of the intervention in the two districts should be comparable to the time-delay between starting the intervention in them.

Thus disparities in timing of similar healthy eating promotion activities in different Health Districts provide opportunities for usefully controlled comparisons. However, if these opportunities are to be taken the different Districts must collect relevant valid data in comparable ways and work together in designing their studies.

Comparisons of self-selected groups within populations

Comparisons of self selected groups within populations compare a group of people who have been exposed to the health promotion activity with a group of people who have not. The investigator however had no control over which person should be in which group. That was decided by the person themselves or by the circumstances of their life. This is the fundamental weakness of this design. We are not sure what determined which group a person should be in and it is possible that it may also influence the variable we are studying. For example if we are trying to promote consumption of vegetables with a programme of leaflets and posters it may be that those who notice our leaflets and posters are those who are more health conscious and if they subsequently increase consumption more than the other group it is because they are more health conscious, not because of our leaflets and posters. In a randomised control study the health consciousness should have been similar in the two groups.

The trick is to think of all the factors (education, income, occupation) likely to interfere with the comparison that we are trying to make and measure them as well. When we come to the data analysis stage we can then make allowance for them and see if they could account for any differences observed. Make sure you will be monitoring the other factors that a sceptic might say were the cause of any difference observed rather than your health promotion.

Comparison of predicted and non-predicted effects (multiple baseline studies)

Health promotion activities aim to produce certain specific changes. They will aim to promote consumption of certain specific foods, to impart certain specific items of knowledge or to influence certain specific attitudes. Comparisons between the specific foods, knowledge or attitudes targeted in the health promotion and the foods, knowledge or attitudes not mentioned can be informative. Differences between targeted and non-targeted variables are most informative when the patterns are in related parts of the cuisine or lifestyle, e.g. total fats and P:S ratio or fish, meats, cheese and eggs. Where the specific targeted item shows changes while closely related but untargeted ones do not this is good evidence that the change in the targeted item was due to the health promotion.

'Message tracking' is a variant of this technique. A 'healthy eating' leaflet might emphasise one type of food, nutrient or eating practice and recall of that advice can be tracked relative to concepts not mentioned in the leaflet. This enables one to see whether any change in behaviour is attributable to these messages.

Comparison of different methods

Another practical but neglected form of comparison is between variants of the same basic activity. Different canteens, corner shops or slimming groups could be given different versions of a handout. Each version should cover the same basic message in equally plausible and practicable ways. Differences in emphasis or selective omission from the different versions allow testing of the relative contribution of different parts of the leaflet.

Of course the same measures must be made of the potential effects of each variant of the leaflet. It is also important wherever practicable to check that attention had been paid to the content of each variant ('manipulation checks') and that each variant was as plausible as the other variants ('believability checks').

Note that unless one variant is markedly less effective than the others, you will not know whether all variants are equally effective or equally ineffective. Also note that this design tests components within the context of that sort of leaflet, and also assumes that components do not depend on each other. The same approach can assess the usefulness of backing up talks with written material (or vice versa), or of different oral or written presentations of the same content, and so on.

Designs without comparison groups

Strictly speaking designs without some sort of comparison group cannot demonstrate cause. There are however two types of study which are commonly used and can provide some rather unreliable evidence for effect of health promotion activity.

The first of these is study of trends. When a predicted change in trend (a 'blip') closely follows an intervention it is tempting to think that the intervention was the cause. For example, suppose sales of skimmed milk from the local stores have been gradually increasing by 3% a month and then in the month immediately after our promotion of the health benefits of skimmed milk they increase by 30% and in the following months they fall back towards the baseline trend. In the absence of other explanations we may suggest that our promotion has caused the increase in purchase of this product. This is very weak evidence but it is better than none.

At the crudest level one can simply measure the item of interest before and immediately after the intervention and assume that any change was due to our activity. For example we could measure knowledge immediately before and immediately after a talk on healthier eating and trust that any change observed in that short time was unlikely to be due to anything else. It is possible that the change might be an effect of repeating the test and it could be that the effect was due to getting together in a group rather than the specific content of the talk. This can only be applied to changes over very short time periods and even then is the weakest sort of evidence.

Further reading

General evaluation theory

Fitz-Gibbon C.T. & Morris L.L. (1987). *How to design a program evaluation* p.168. Sage, London
Nutbeam D., Smith C. & Catford J. (1990). 'Evaluation in health education: a review of progress and possibilities.'
Journal of Epidemiology and Community Health 44, 83-89.

Example of random control design

MRFIT Research Group (1982). 'Multiple Risk Factor Intervention Trial: Risk factor changes and mortality results.'
Journal of American Medical Association 248, 1465-1477.
Nichols S., Waters W.E., Woolaway M. & Hamilton Smith M. (1988). 'Evaluation of the effectiveness of a nutritional health education leaflet in changing public knowledge and attitudes.'
Journal of Human Nutrition and Dietetics 1, 233-238.
Fehily A., Vaughan-Williams E., Shiels K. and five others (1989). 'The effect of dietary advice on nutrient intakes. Evidence from the diet and reinfarction trial.'
Journal of Human Nutrition and Dietetics 2, 225-235.

Examples of group comparision design

Puska P., Tuomlehlo J., Salonen J., and six others (1979). 'Changes in coronary risk factors during the comprehensive five year community programme to control cardiovascular disease.'
British Medical Journal 2, 1173-1178.

Walter H.J., Hofman A., Vaughan R.D. & Wynder E.L. (1988). 'Modification risk factors for coronary heart disease – five year result of a school-based intervention trial.'
New England Journal of Medicine 318, 1093-1100.

Example of comparison of self-selected groups

Charny M. & Lewis P.A. (1987). 'Does health knowledge affect eating habits?'
Health Education Journal 46, 172-176.

Watson D., Moreton W. & Jessop E.G. (1988). 'Coronary awareness. Evaluation of weeks' campaign.'
Health Education Journal 47, 49-53.

5 · What is meant by validation?

Summary

Results must be valid and reproducible. A valid procedure is one which really measures what it is supposed to measure. Validity has several aspects including face validity, content validity, criterion validity and construct validity. The meaning of each of these and ways of assessing them are described.

Introduction

This chapter deals with some fundamental theory of measurement. You may want to skip it in your first reading of the book. However the question of validity is of crucial importance and the subject matter covered in this chapter must be considered before you set about any study.

Once you have decided what information you want to collect the next problem is deciding how to collect it. You will want to be sure that the information you produce is correct and you will also need to be able to convince other people that your information is correct.

Methods of collecting information

If we want to know how much salt someone adds to their food there are several different methods we could use to obtain this information. We could talk with them about their eating habits, steering the conversation to cover use of salt in various circumstances; this method of collecting data is called an interview. We could read out a list of questions about use of salt and record the answers or we could write the questions down and get the respondents to write down their answers; these methods are called an interview administered questionnaire and a self-administered questionnaire. We could in principle follow the person round and unobtrusively record every situation in which they used salt (and possibly weigh the salt pot before and after they used it to estimate how much salt they had used); this would be called an observation of behaviour. Lastly we could ask them to make a record of their salt use.

The different ways of collecting information are summarised in Table 5.1.

Table 5.1   Methods of collecting information about people

Unstructured interview
Semi-structured interview
Group discussion
Interview administered questionnaire
Self-administered questionnaire
Self-recorded behaviour
Observation of behaviour

What is an instrument?

Survey workers talk about measurement 'instruments' by which they mean any device for measuring something. A simple question is an 'instrument' but an instrument could equally well be a group of questions or a long questionnaire or an interview or an observation of behaviour or the use of a machine. In this chapter we will use the example of the question and answer method to explain what is meant by validity, but the same principles can just as well be applied to any other measurement instrument.

What is validity?

Whatever method we choose we have to consider the validity of the results we obtain by using it. The word 'validity' is used to describe the ability of a measurement procedure to really measure whatever it is that we are trying to measure. A measurement procedure is 'valid' if we can rule out all interpretations of the result other than the one that we have placed upon it. Definitions of validity are given in Box 5.1. The definitions of the different types of validity are not agreed by everyone and you may find slightly different definitions of validity in some books.

In the situation where a group of workers are deeply committed to a project you will need to be sure of your ground before saying that it has failed to meet its objectives. Similarly in a situation where management is keen to close down a project you will require very solid evidence that the project is producing good results to dissuade them. These two examples describe conflict situations where it is obviously vital that your information is correct and can be shown to be correct. However validity is no less important in other situations. It means that your result can be relied upon and your claims are really true.

A simple example

Suppose we are discussing meals in the hospital canteen. One person says 'I
interviewed 100 people. Only 15% said they usually ate lunch in the canteen and
only 10% said that they thought canteen meals were good', while someone else
says 'That's rubbish – 100 people filled in a written questionnaire for me and
85% said they usually ate lunch in the canteen and 90% said they thought that
canteen meals were good'. How do we decide which if any report to believe?
Were the results of the first person, or the results of the second, the more valid?

65

Who was the sample?

The first question to be settled is who were the 100 people contacted by the two observers? Were they similar groups and were both groups representative of hospital staff? For the sake of this argument we will assume that the two observers interviewed the same 100 people so that sampling cannot account for the difference in their conclusions. The whole question of how we select people (sampling) for study is very important and will be covered in Chapter 7.

What are you trying to measure?

The first step in measuring anything is deciding exactly what it is that we are trying to measure. We cannot begin to assess validity until this has been decided. In our simple example the phrase 'thinking canteen meals good' is confusing and does not make clear what it was that the investigators were trying to study. We will assume that what they were really trying to measure was how far people judge canteen meals to be close to what they would most like.

Face validity

The next thing to establish is exactly what questions were asked and how they were asked. In our example the first question was presumably 'When you are at work where do you usually eat lunch?'. On the face of it this would seem a reasonable way of finding out whether they eat in the hospital canteen and so the question has 'face validity'. The questions about what they thought about the quality of canteen meals is more difficult. If for example we find out that the question was 'What do you think of hospital catering?' then subjects may well have been confused as to whether it referred to meals for patients or staff. Such a question would have poor face validity.

The face validity of a question is also affected by the way and the situation in which it is asked. The next chapter describes how to ask or write questions in a valid fashion. Generally we try and make the face validity of a question as good as possible in two ways. First we ask people who know a great deal about the topic that we wish to investigate what they think about the question. Second we ask the sorts of people whom we wish to answer the question to check that they understand the question in the way that was intended.

Content validity

The next approach we must use is to ask the question 'Does the result obtained with our question really represent the skill, belief, value or behaviour that we are trying to measure?'. The first problem is that it may be very difficult to explain exactly what it is that we are trying to measure. 'Usually eating lunch in the canteen' is easy to explain (though the vague word 'usually' may cause difficulty). An earlier section discussed the concept underlying 'thinking the canteen meals good' and decided that it was concerned with how close people felt canteen meals were to what they wanted. It is thus a composite of people's judgements on the taste, appearance, healthiness and value for money of the meals.

Content validity is whether the question covers all aspects of what we are trying to measure. We have seen that the general idea of 'thinking canteen meals good' has several aspects. A question such as 'do you think canteen meals taste good?' on the other hand only covers part of what people want and misses out other important aspects such as value for money, appearance and healthiness. This question therefore has poor 'content validity' because it only partially covers the characteristic that we are trying to measure.

Construct validity

Construct validity asks whether in a situation where we think we know what to expect, the question gives us the results we expect. For example we might expect (make the hypothesis) that people who work evening shifts and therefore are not in the hospital at lunchtime would be less likely to eat lunch in the canteen. If we look at the results and find no difference in answers between those working evenings and those working daytime, that would suggest that there was something wrong with the question and it has poor 'construct validity'.

Similarly we might expect that people who think canteen meals are good will be more likely to eat their lunch in the canteen. We could show 'construct validity' of the question on 'thinking canteen catering good' by showing that people who eat lunch in the canteen are more likely to say that they think the catering good than people who never eat in the canteen. If we do not get this expected result it may be because the question has poor 'construct validity'. It could also be because the information on who usually eats in the canteen is wrong or because our original expectation was wrong. (Maybe people who do not eat in the canteen do not realise that the catering is awful!)

Another test of the construct validity of the question on 'thinking canteen catering good' could be made if we improved the catering arrangements. If under these circumstances the proportion of people rating the catering as good did not increase then the question is not producing construct valid responses (or we have failed in our attempts to improve the attractiveness of the catering).

Criterion validity

We may be able to settle the question of what proportion of people ate hospital lunches by looking at a different source of information. If we approach the catering manager he might tell us that he usually sells 700 lunches and we know that the hospital has 1000 employees. This would suggest that on the question of the percentage of staff who eat lunch in the canteen the second report gives the better estimate (assuming the sales record is accurate and most people eat only one lunch).

This is an example of validating a question by comparing it with another method which is generally believed to be correct and is based on different assumptions. Validity shown in this way is called 'criterion validity' or sometimes 'concurrent validity'. It is not foolproof because both methods could agree but give the wrong answer. Unfortunately we frequently do not have a 'gold standard' measurement or even any alternative measurement to compare our instrument with. For example we had no such convenient way of testing the validity of the estimates of how many people thought canteen meals were good.

There are various ways of measuring the criterion validity of an instrument which are shown in Boxes 5.2 and 5.3.

Box 5.2

Criterion validation of a measure of a nominal* variable

Suppose we wished to test the validity of a question intended to decide whether people were intolerant of tartrazine. The question is 'Are you allergic to tartrazine?'.

For our criterion method we will give each person four apparently identical orange drinks on four different days, two of which contain large doses of tartrazine and two do not. We will carefully enquire whether the subject had any symptoms after each test and classify those who had symptoms after the tartrazine drinks as 'truly' allergic. (Many people would argue that this is not an appropriate criterion but for this example we will assume it produces the true answer.)

The responses to the question and the challenge test can then be shown as follows:

		Challenge Test		
		Reaction	No reaction	
Answer to	Yes	20	20	40
Question	No	5	55	60
		25	75	

We can see that there is not perfect agreement between the question and the criterion method. Half of those who answer 'yes' to the question do not react to the challenge test and five who answer 'no' do react.

Continued opposite

Box 5.2 (Continued)

We can measure the degree of agreement by sensitivity and specificity.

		Criterion Method	
		Positive	*Negative*
Method being validated	*Positive*	True Positive	False Positive
	Negative	False Negative	True Negative

$$\text{Sensitivity} = \frac{\text{True positives}}{\text{True positives} + \text{False negatives}}$$

$$\text{Specificity} = \frac{\text{True negatives}}{\text{True negatives} + \text{False positives}}$$

A sensitivity of 1 indicates that the method correctly identifies all positives. A specificity of 1 indicates that the method correctly identifies all negatives. A low specificity or sensitivity indicates that the test does no better than chance (i.e. tossing a coin would give equally correct results).

Note the sensitivity and specificity of an instrument will depend not only on the instrument itself but also on the frequency of true positives in the group being studied.

*A nominal variable is one where each value represents a different group. In this example the variable 'allergy to tartrazine' has only two possible values 'allergic' and 'not allergic'. Other examples of nominal variables are sex (male and female), place of residence or ethnic group. See Box 6.2 for explanation of types of data.

Box 5.3

Criterion validation of ratio* variable

A questionnaire has been developed which is intended to measure salt intake. The most reliable measure of salt intake is probably urinary sodium excretion. Twenty four hour urinary sodium excretion has therefore been used as the criterion method. The test group of subjects completed the questionnaire and made a series of 24-hour urine collections which were analysed for sodium content. The results are shown below.

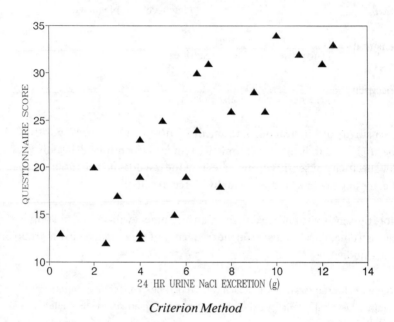

Criterion Method

It can be seen that the two estimates (questionnaire score and 24-hour urine sodium excretion) agree fairly well. The agreement between the two estimates is measured by the correlation coefficient (written as r). A correlation coefficient of 1 or − 1 indicates perfect agreement; a correlation coefficient of 0 indicates no agreement.

*Salt intake is an example of a ratio variable. Other examples are body weight, plasma cholesterol level and income. Ratio variables are continuous and their properties are further explained in Box 6.2.

Reproducibility

Allied to validity is the question of reproducibility. Reproducibility is sometimes also called reliability. If we ask the same person the question several times, do we get the same answer each time? The obvious way of checking reproducibility is to ask the same person the same question on more than one occasion in circumstances where the answer should not change. However memory is liable to inflate this estimate of reliability. Alternatively we can check reproducibility by asking the same question of two different but similar samples taken from the same population. Poor reproducibility is a sign of poor validity but good reproducibility does not necessarily mean good validity. A question may produce very reproducible results but they may be consistently wrong. The connection between reproducibility and validity is explained further in Box 5.4.

There are all sorts of reasons why a question may have poor reproducibility and Box 5.5 lists the various sources of variation. Good technique of setting and asking questions as explained in the next chapter will improve reproducibility.

Validation in different populations

Just because an instrument has been shown to be valid and reproducible in one population you cannot assume that it will be valid and reproducible in a different population. An instrument developed and validated in America may not be valid in England; an instrument developed and validated in Birmingham may not be valid in Stoke or Coventry; and an instrument developed for use in a prosperous suburb may not be valid in a deprived inner city district.

Box 5.4

The relationship of reproducibility and validity

Criterion validity is measured by the correlation between the method being validated and the reference method. The maximum correlation possible is limited by the reproducibility of the two measures.

The relationship is given by the following formula:
$$rmax_{ab} = \sqrt{R_a \cdot R_b}$$
Where $rmax_{ab}$ is maximum possible correlation between methods a and b
R_a and R_b are reproducibilities for methods a and b.

Box 5.5

Sources of variation

There are a number of reasons why we do not get the same answer each time we repeat a measurement on the same subject. These are called sources of variation.

1 *Real difference*
   The actual state of the subject may have changed between two measurements.

2 *Error*
   Error (difference from the 'true' value) is an important cause of variation but not all variation is due to error.

   There are two main types of error:
   1 Systematic error – a value which differs from the 'true' value in a constant direction (systematically) i.e. always overestimates or always underestimates.
   2 Random error – a value which differs from the 'true' value but is just as likely to overestimate as to underestimate.

Sources of error

1 *Inter-observer and intra-observer*
   If the measurements are made by different observers they may use slightly different techniques (inter-observer variation). If the measurement is made on both occasions by the same observer they may use slightly different techniques each time (intra-observer variation). These two sources of variation may be reduced by carefully defining what it is that we are trying to measure and by rigidly standardising procedures of measurement.

2 *Instrument variation*
   Variation can arise from the instrument (e.g. questionnaire, interview method, weighing scales, cholesterol analyser). Instrument variation is basically of two types:
   (a) Zero error – variation in the zero setting of the instrument
   (b) Range error – variation in the measurement of differences in value

   Instrument variation is minimised by careful calibration of instruments.

Further reading

General discussion of validity

Chapters 7 and 8 of Abramson J. H. (1984)
  Survey Methods in Community Medicine – 3rd Edition – Churchill Livingstone,
  Edinburgh.
Chapter 2 of McDowell I. & Newell C. (1987). *Measuring Health*:
  A Guide to Rating Scales and Questionnaires. Oxford University Press, Oxford.

Validity related to food consumption

Chapters 9 and 10 of Cameron M. E. & Van Staveren W. A. (1980).
  Manual on methodology for food consumption studies. Oxford University
  Press, Oxford.

6 · Interviews and questionnaires

Summary

The advantages and disadvantages of interviewing and self-completion questionnaires are compared. Good interviewing is a difficult skill and the chapter gives a short description of the principles of interviewing.

The next section deals with principles of questionnaire design. It includes the characteristics of good and bad questions, whether to use open or closed questions and how to set responses for closed questions. Developing valid questions and methods for yourself is difficult and time consuming. You should consider the advantages of using published methods developed by other people.

Introduction

The previous chapter listed the different ways of collecting information (Table 5.1) and then explained why it was so important to ensure that, whatever method you choose, the instruments you use are valid. This chapter explains how to ensure validity of measurements made with two of the most widely used methods.

Principles of interviewing

Types of interview

Interviews involve collecting information through talking to someone (the interviewee) and listening to and recording their responses. Interviews may be administered face to face or over the telephone. There are many different ways of doing this.

An unstructured interview is very like a natural conversation in which the interviewee is encouraged to describe their experiences and to express their views. Only the broad topic is decided before an unstructured interview. The questions asked and the order in which they are asked depends on the topics raised by the interviewee and on the ways in which the interviewer tries to keep the conversation going.

For a fully structured interview the questions to be asked, their precise wording, and the order in which they are to be asked are all decided before the interview. The interviewer may be required to ask supplementary questions (prompts) but the nature and wording of these prompts and the circumstances in which they are to be used are also decided before the interview. A questionnaire administered by an interviewer is an example of a fully structured interview.

The semi-structured interview is a compromise between the fully structured and the unstructured interview methods. The interviewer will have a list of questions on which they wish to obtain the views of the interviewee but will incorporate these at more or less appropriate moments during the interview. The precise way in which the questions are asked and sometimes the order in which they are asked are determined by the flow of the conversation.

Taking a 'dietary history' or a 'clinical history' are special forms of semi-structured interviewing.

Group discussion may be considered to be a special variant of the interview method. Here a small number of people are invited to discuss a topic of interest while the leader steers the discussion so as to bring out the participants' views of that topic. A tape recording and transcript is made or at least key points are noted down to provide a permanent record.

Interviewing skills

The skill of a good interviewer is to draw out all the information without introducing bias. This involves having a pleasant manner so that people feel ready to give information. The interviewer has to prompt the interviewee to expand on topics of particular interest without indicating a preference for any particular response. They must not suggest by tone of voice, by facial expression or by any other way that they approve or disapprove of any response. This requirement for unbiased information may make it very difficult for a care giver also to act as information collector. (For example the interviewer may feel that it is unwise for an interviewee to dine off pork pies and ten pints of beer each night but if they are trying to collect information in an unbiased way they must appear totally neutral to this information.)

The interviewer must record the result of the interview so that the information obtained from the record later accurately reflects the interviewee's views and opinions. The use of properly organised recording forms will be helpful.

Advantages and disadvantages of interviewing

The advantage of unstructured interviewing is that it is very flexible and allows you to follow up leads and to collect information on topics you may not have thought of. Face-to-face interaction or tone of voice gives some assurance that the interviewee is responding seriously and trying to give accurate replies. It may also seem the easiest method to collect information. In reality unstructured interviewing is a very difficult skill and structured interviewing has to satisfy all the requirements of good questionnaire design discussed in the next section.

The disadvantage of interviewing (especially an unstructured interview) is that it often has low validity. It is very difficult to avoid observer bias. Two unskilled interviewers can interview the same person and come back with completely different impressions of their views. The risk is always present that the interviewees gives the response that they think the interviewer wants to hear rather than their real response. Of course data collected by interview cannot be totally anonymous. The pitfalls of interviewing are well recognised among opinion pollsters and market researchers. Any reputable research organisation will insist that all its interviewers have at least basic training in interview skills.

Generally the less structured interview method is best suited to preliminary investigations or when you want to collect information from one or two people (e.g. what the two Catering Managers in your district think about healthier eating). The interview method is also well suited for 'in-depth' studies of what a few people feel about a certain aspect of eating or of health.

Principles of questionnaire design

Requirements of a good question

The characteristics of a good question written or spoken are listed in Table 6.1.

Table 6.1

Requirements of a good question

Clear and unambiguous
Free from bias
Not offensive
Contains only one idea
Appropriate level of difficulty
Easy to use answer format
Face validity

The questions have to be clear and unambiguous so that everyone understands them to mean the same. 'Do you usually have a drink with your dinner?' is a bad question. Some respondents may call their midday meal dinner while others call their evening meal dinner. It is also unclear whether you mean just alcoholic drinks or whether you are also interested in glasses of water and cups of tea. The question 'Have you had any of the following symptoms after eating food? – headaches, abdominal pains, palpitations, nasal congestion or rhinorrhoea' needs to have all the medical jargon removed and to be turned into everyday English so that people can understand it.

The question must be free from bias so that the respondent (the person answering the question) is not led into giving a particular answer. Consider the question 'How many times in the last year have you had to go without a meal because you were short of money?'. This question is bad because it clearly suggests that it expects you to have missed meals because of shortage of money. It would be much better asked as two questions 'In the past year have you ever had to miss a meal because of shortage of money?'. Those who said yes could then be asked 'How many times has this happened?'. Another example of a biased question is 'Do you think additives and other toxic chemicals should be used in school meals?'.

Questions should not be offensive. Questions such as 'Do you give your children unhealthy food?' and 'Would you say that you were fat?' are bad because they may well suggest to the respondent that you have a low opinion of them.

Generally each question should contain only one idea. The question 'If you think how you eat affects the risk of heart disease, what changes have you made in your diet?' is thoroughly confusing and the answers you might get would be uninterpretable. It would be much better asked as several questions. 'Have you made any changes in your diet in the past year?' 'If so what were these changes?' 'For each change what was your reason for making it?' and lastly 'Do you think that how you eat affects your risk of heart disease?'.

Questions also need to be of appropriate difficulty for the respondents. There is little point in asking a question such as 'How many grammes of carbohydrate would you say you ate in a day?' in a shopper's survey because most of them would not have a clue what you were talking about. On the other hand this might be a reasonable question for patients attending a diabetic clinic. Similarly there would be little point in including a question such as 'Do you think short chain saturated fatty acids are less atherogenic than long chain saturated fatty acids?' in a general survey though it could be a useful question in a survey of cardiologists.

When developing questions you should ask yourself whether each question meets all these requirements. Then seek the opinions of colleagues who may see ambiguities and other problems you have missed. Finally try them out with a few people like those with whom you intend to use the questions, consider their answers and ask them what they think of the questions.

Open or closed questions

Both interview-administered questionnaires and self-completed questionnaires can be divided into open-ended and closed questions. 'What do you think of the food served to you in hospital?' is an example of an open-ended question. 'Would you say the food served to you in hospital was (i) good or (ii) adequate or (iii) poor?' is an example of a closed question.

Open-ended questions have the advantage of allowing the respondent to provide more information than closed questions. For example one patient may reply to

---

Box 6.1

Comparison of open and closed questions

	Open	*Closed*
Information content	As much as respondent is prepared to give. May be very rich May be poor	Limited
Likelihood of unexpected response	Probable	Negligible
Likelihood of response requirement being misinterpreted	More likely	Less likely
Ease of completion	May be difficult	Very easy
Need for respondent co-operation	Needs high co-operation	Needs little co-operation
Ease of coding responses	Difficult	Very easy
Ease of grouping responses	Difficult	Very easy
Possibility of changing response grouping	Can be done	Cannot be done
Difficulty of designing questions	Less difficult	More difficult
Summary	Sometimes very informative but demanding for respondent and awkward to process	Less informative, less demanding for respondent and easy to process.

---

the open question that the food was 'absolutely awful and looked revolting' while another might say that it was 'eatable but not very exciting'. Clearly these patients have different opinions but both might have chosen the same response of 'poor' to the closed question. Another patient might reply to the open question 'generally very good, well cooked and tasty but the portions were rather small'. This is much more informative than the response of 'good' which he would have given to the closed question.

On the other hand patients may give ambiguous responses to open-ended questions. The open question might produce a response like 'O.K.' which is not very informative. Other possible responses such as 'My mother's cooking is better' or 'The custard is lumpy' are difficult to categorise.

The relative advantages and disadvantages of each type of question are summarised in Box 6.1. The advantages of closed questions are that they may be easier to answer quickly, there is less scope for misunderstanding the question and the responses will be easier to process. Generally closed questions are better for surveys where you want to obtain information from large numbers of people quickly, and perhaps for postal surveys.

Open questions are particularly useful in the early stages of developing a survey instrument when you are not sure what responses to expect. It is also a good idea to include an open question such as 'Is there anything else you would like to say about the healthier eating exhibition?' at the end of a set of closed questions.

Setting responses in closed questions

Considerable care is required in choosing response categories for closed questions. There has to be a category for every possible response and if only one response is allowed then each respondent must fit into only one of the categories.

Consider the question:

'How often do you eat breakfast cereal?

A   Less than once a week
B   1-3 times a week
C   3-5 times a week
D   Every day
E   More than once a day'

Which answer do I give if I eat cereal three times a week (B or C)? Which answer do I select if I eat cereal six times a week?

Or consider this question:

'Which of these do you think are the most important causes of heart disease?

A Smoking
B Eating fatty foods
C Fluoride in water
D Smoking and eating fatty foods
E All of these'

Which answer do I select if I think that none of them are important? Which do I select if I think that smoking and fluoride in water but not fatty foods are important? These difficulties could be avoided by resetting the question in the following form:

'Do you think these are important causes of heart disease? (You may say yes to more than one if you wish.)

A	Smoking	Yes	No
B	Eating fatty foods	Yes	No
C	Fluoride in drinking water	Yes	No'

Note also that this question allows us to distinguish someone who thinks none of the suggested causes is important (all responses No) and someone who failed to answer the question (all responses blank). If we had merely asked people to tick the causes they thought important we could not have made this distinction. It is good practice to design questions so that there is no possibility of making a valid blank response.

Often it is necessary to include a response such as 'other – please specify' or 'don't know' or 'not applicable' to ensure that there is a possible response for everyone.

Response categories have to be chosen so as not to introduce bias. Generally the number of favourable and unfavourable responses should be equal and the extremes should be equally strong. The following question illustrates how clumsy setting of response categories can introduce bias:

'What phrase best describes your attitude to heart disease?

A Not worried
B Slightly worried
C Very worried
D Extremely worried'

Usually (but not always) we want to set our categories so as to divide the respondents into equal size groups. It is therefore helpful to have a rough idea of the likely frequency of responses before deciding how to set the response categories.

The order of questions

Once the questions have been decided it is necessary to arrange them in an appropriate order. They should be in a logical order so that there is a natural flow of ideas from question to question. Sometimes asking one question will affect the answer to another one. For example the question 'Do you think eating fried foods increases your risk of heart disease?' may affect the response to the question 'How often do you give your children fried foods?'. The question on how often should be placed before the question on risk of heart disease.

Some questions may be considered sensitive and these should generally come at the end of the questionnaire. 'How old are you?', 'Are you married?', 'What is your income?', 'How much do you spend on alcohol?' are examples of questions which may be sensitive. If these questions have to be asked the response categories (i.e. age group, income band) should be the broadest which are still useful.

Piloting

You will have gathered from Chapter 5 that producing valid questions or other instruments is not an easy task. It requires many hours of thought and discussion. When you think you have got the questions ready, you will have to try them out (pilot them). Next you have to use the information gained from this try-out to alter and improve the questions before trying them out again.

When at long last you think you have got the questions right you should try and show that they are face valid, content valid, construct valid, criterion valid and reproducible.

Dimensions, scales and items

At this stage we must introduce three more technical words 'dimensions', 'scales' and 'items'. So far we have talked about questions and how they can be used to 'measure' something. We are therefore making the assumption that there is an underlying quantity of something which we can estimate from our answers. The something we are trying to estimate is called a dimension. Examples of the dimensions whose quantities we might try to estimate are frequency of eating cabbage, amount of fat consumed, strength of liking for chocolate and strength of belief in preventability of heart disease. This process of estimating underlying quantity from responses to questions is called scaling. Each question constitutes an 'item' and there are single item scales (based on one question) and multi item scales (based on more than one question). Good scales should estimate a single dimension but all too frequently several different dimensions get muddled up in one single score obtained from a set of different questions.

Types of scales

The different types of scale can best be understood by considering some closed response questions:

What do you usually spread on your bread?

a) Butter   b) Margarine   c) Other spreads

The responses to this question are not graded and are an example of nominal data or a list in no particular order. (These are also called categorical scales.) All we can say is that people who eat margarine differ in this respect from those who eat butter, we cannot put them in order or calculate a population average.

How thickly do you spread your bread with butter or margarine?

a) Thinly   b) Medium   c) Thickly

How many slices of bread do you usually eat in a day?

a) 0   b) 1   c) 2   d) 3   e) 4   f) 5   g) 6 or more

These two responses are examples of different types of graded data. The first set of responses may form an ordinal scale and the second a ratio scale (except for category g). In both types we can place the responses in order. However we can calculate population averages and perform other arithmetical manipulations on ratio type scales but not on ordinal type scales. You will find more information on types of scale in Box 6.2. The ways of presenting the different types of data are discussed in Chapter 16.

Multi-item scales

So far we have considered only single questions but often several questions are used to measure one attribute (or dimension). Suppose we wished to measure liking for fried food; we might use four questions:

Box 6.2

Types of Data (Scale)

1 Nominal Data

Definition: A nominal scale is one where the classes are mutually exclusive, but have no intrinsic order or value.

Examples: 1   Sex (male/female)

             2   The International Classification of Diseases (ICD)
This lists all the diseases it is possible to die from – nearly one thousand of them. (Note that there have to be strict rules for classifying people who happen to have two or more diseases concurrently.)

             3   We could classify fruit:
Apples, Pears, Oranges, Bananas, Other;
or vegetables:
Green leaf veg., Root veg., Green legumes, Squashes, Other.

Nominal data have no particular order
The fruit and vegetable lists could have been written in any order at all (except perhaps for putting 'Other' at the end), and it would not have changed your understanding of what was being done. There is no sense in which 'Apple' is better than, more worthy than, or takes precedence over, 'Orange'.

Classification systems used in nominal 'scales' or any other scale type must be:

        mutually exclusive
        i.e. a vegetable cannot simultaneously be green leaf and root;

        exhaustive
        The 'Other' category ensures that *all* fruit and vegetables can be classified somewhere. Even the ICD had what amounts to an 'Other' category;

Presentation: Nominal data can only be presented as frequencies of occurrence.

Continued opposite

Box 6.2 (Continued)

2 Ordinal Data

Definition: An ordinal 'scale' is one where the classes can be placed in order (e.g. 'is bigger than' or 'is preferred to'), but in which the amount by which one is bigger than or preferred to another is not specified.

Examples: 1 Response categories of how people behave or feel are often of this kind;

  e.g. 'As compared with last year are you drinking? (Ring one response)

Much more	More	About the same	Less	Much less'

Frequently, numbers are used to label ordinal scale points, e.g. 5, 4, 3, 2, 1. These numbers are arbitrary labels bearing an *ordered* relationship to each other, but not one of magnitude. The difference between responses 3 and 2 is not necessarily the same as the difference between responses 5 and 4.

  2 Degrees of agreement can form ordinal data e.g. 'Fats are bad for the heart (Ring one response)

Strongly agree	Agree	Neither agree nor disagree	Disagree	Strongly disagree'

  3 Orders of preference of foods and other rankings can reflect measurement on an ordinal scale.

  4 Social class (I, II, III non-manual, III manual, IV, V) is sometimes treated as an ordinal data. (See Box 2.3)

Presentation: Ordinal data must be treated as ranks and not as scores. They must not be averaged or otherwise arithmetically manipulated.

3 Interval Data

Interval scales are only included here for the sake of completeness and it is unlikely that you will need to use one.

Definition: An interval scale is one where the data points are ordered and the size of the difference between data points is specified but the scale has no absolute zero so that the ratio of one point to another is not specified.

One of the few examples of an interval scale is Centigrade or Farenheit temperature ($2°C$ is not twice at hot as $1°C$ nor $-1°$ half as hot as $-2°C$).

Continued overleaf

'Please state how much you like the following:

1	Fried eggs	Like very much	Like	Dislike	Dislike very much
2	Fried sausage	Like very much	Like	Dislike	Dislike very much
3	Fried fish	Like very much	Like	Dislike	Dislike very much
4	Fried bacon	Like very much	Like	Dislike	Dislike very much'

The answers to these four questions (or items) might then be shown to be combinable to form a multi-item scale measuring 'Liking for fried food'.

Combining the responses from different items to form a single multi-item score is only legitimate if the response to each of the items is largely influenced by the same attribute (i.e. they all measure the same dimension). We can tell whether the different items really measure a single dimension by looking at the relation of the different answers to each other. If the different items do not behave like a single dimension any multi-item score made by combining them will be meaningless.

In choosing items in the hope of making up a multi-item scale it is also important that the questions cover most of the dimension you are trying to measure. In the 'liking for fried foods' example we would want to be sure that these four foods were representative of the fried foods with which the respondent was familiar.

Once we have chosen items that seem appropriate to use and have some reason for thinking that the different items can be combined to form a multi-item scale, the next problem is how to combine them. It is safe to assume that someone who answers 'dislike very much' to all four questions likes fried food less than someone who answers 'like very much' to all four. However, does someone who 'dislikes very much' fried fish and fried bacon but 'likes' fried eggs and fried sausage like fried food more or less than someone who 'likes very much' fried fish but 'dislikes very much' the other three fried foods? This simple example shows some of the problems in constructing and scoring multi-item scales.

In order to combine the items we have to do two things. First, we have to convert the individual items into a data type which can be combined (convert from ordinal to ratio data – see Box 6.2). Second, we have to devise valid rules for combining the item scores into a unidimensional score.

Multi-item scores are very commonly used. Knowledge scores and healthy eating scores are examples of multi-item scores. Genuine multi-item scales are difficult to develop and validate. If you are contemplating trying to construct one you certainly ought to discuss it with a statistician. There is further discussion of multi-item scales and some guidance on how to construct your own in Box 6.3.

Should you develop your own instrument or use someone else's?

One of the reasons for writing this guide was the feeling that a lot of effort is wasted in the Health Service by using badly designed instruments in badly designed studies. If we shared experience and tried to use only a few well validated and reproducible instruments we might do a lot better.

The advantage of developing your own instrument is that you should be able to collect exactly the information you want. The disadvantages are that you will have to spend a lot of time developing and validating the instrument. Even then because of limitation of expertise, time and resource you are liable to end up with one which has doubtful validity and reproducibility. Certainly, before deciding to make your own questionnaire or other measurement instrument, you ought to find out what ones are already available and have good reasons for not using them.

A further disadvantage of using your own instrument is that it means it will be difficult to compare your results with results obtained using other instruments. If it appears that your District is different from the next door District (for example, fewer people eat wholemeal bread or people are less concerned about

Box 6.3

Constructing your own multi-item scales

1 Do the items lie on a single dimension?
The basic indication that items lie on different dimensions is *low* correlation.

2 Collecting data to use in constructing a multi-item scale
Collect answers to your set of items from five times as many people as you have items (i.e. if you have ten items you should have answers from at least 50 people). The people you get to answer the questions should be similar to the target population on whom you hope to use the scale eventually.

3. Scoring the items
Each scale point on each item must be scored (given a numeric value).
A dichotomous item has two responses (e.g. True/False, Eats/Does not eat, Agrees/Disagrees) which may be scored as 0 and 1.
Items with more than two response categories (e.g. Strongly agree, Agree, Disagree, Strongly disagree) must be given a value for each points. In this example the points could be given values of $+3, +1, -1, -3$.
N.B. This is converting ordinal data into an interval data and involves some very risky assumptions that should be checked by scaling the data.

4 Compiling the correlation matrix
Calculate the correlations between all possible pairs of items. The type of correlation coefficient to be calculated depends on what sort of items you are using and the response patterns obtained. The use of an appropriate statistical package on a micro-computer makes calculation of correlation coefficients a relatively easy task.

Consider the 'Liking for fried foods' example given in the text. There were four items: Eggs, Sausages, Fish and Bacon. This gives six possible item pairs Eggs-Sausage, Eggs-Fish, Eggs-Bacon, Sausages-Fish, Sausages-Bacon and Fish-Bacon for each of which you must calculate the correlations between people's responses.

The correlation coefficients might be laid out in a matrix like this:

	Sausages	Fish	Bacon
Eggs	0.78	0.24	0.97
Sausages		-0.32	0.83
Fish			-0.43

Correlations ($+$ or $-$) above 0.7 suggest it is reasonable to include the items in the same multi-item score but correlations below 0.5 suggest that they should not be included in the same score.

Continued opposite

Box 6.3 (Continued)

The matrix shown would be reasonable evidence that eggs, sausage and bacon lie on a single dimension of liking for fried foods and can be used to form a scale. Fish lies on a different dimension and therefore should not be included in the same multi-item score as the other three foods.

5 Adding the items to make a multi-item scale
The simplest way to combine items in a multi-item score is to add the component response scores.

This is a rough and ready way to construct a multi-item score but is probably adequate for most purposes.

6 Weightings
Simple addition of scores implies that all items are of equal importance since all contribute equally to the multi-item scale score. Where some items are felt to be more important than others they may be weighted (i.e. their score is multiplied by a number so that it counts more). Statistical procedures can be used to calculate appropriate weightings.

Some statistical procedures for constructing scales

A. Factor Analysis or Principal Component Analysis
These procedures identify mathematical factors underlying the correlations between items and can be used to construct scales and subscales from multi-item questionnaires or any other set of measures.

B. Discriminant Analysis
If you want to produce a multi-item scale that discriminates between different groups then discriminant analysis can be used to optimise the discriminatory power of the scale.

Get Help!
If you are worried about how to use a multiple measure discuss it with a statistician or other person who knows about the subtleties of multi-item scales.

---

heart disease) is that a real difference or is it only because you used different instruments to collect the information?

Even if you take a well validated and widely used instrument you do not entirely avoid the need for validation. As explained in Chapter 5 an instrument should be validated each time it is used in a different population. You should always try and show that the instrument you are using is valid in the particular circumstances in which you are using it.

Modifying an existing instrument

You may decide to compromise by taking a ready developed questionnaire and then modifying it to suit your own particular interest. This may be a good idea but beware! A published questionnaire will have been validated in the form published and quite minor changes may destroy its validity. In particular, changing the wording of questions is likely to ruin their validity. Certainly a multi-item score is likely to become meaningless unless you use all the items in their original form and with the original answer format that was scaled.

Even changing the order of questions is dangerous. For example, consider a validated questionnaire on how often people drink alcohol. If you place a series of questions on attitudes to alcohol abuse before the questions on how often alcohol is drunk you may completely alter the responses given to these. In general, adding extra questions on to the end is the least dangerous way of modifying an existing questionnaire.

If you take an existing instrument and alter it unwisely you may end up with the worst of both worlds. It does not give you the information in which you are most interested because it was developed for some other purpose and yet it is thoroughly invalid because you have mucked it about.

Further reading

Questionnaire design

McDowell I. & Newell C. (1987). *Measuring Health*: *A Guide to Rating Scales and Questionnaires*. Oxford University Press, New York and Oxford.

Bradurn N. N. & Sudmore S. (1979).
Improving Interview Method and Questionnaire Design. Jossey-Bass, San Francisco.

Ratio scaling of questionnaire responses

Child D. (1990). *The Essentials of Factor Analysis*: Chapter 5. Some Applications. Holt, Rinehard & Wilson, London.

Cronbach L. J. (1984). *Essentials of Psychological Testing*: Harper & Row.

7 · Taking a sample

by T. Marshall

Summary

Usually we cannot study everyone in the group (population) of interest to us and we have to draw a sample. It is important that this sample should be representative of the group from which it is drawn.

Random sampling is the preferred method of ensuring an unbiased selection. The two simplest methods are simple random sampling and quasi random sampling. Stratified random sampling is often used to ensure better representativeness. More complex sampling methods which have the merit of simplifying fieldwork are also available.

All random sampling procedures require a sampling frame, i.e. a complete list of population from which the sample will be chosen. Where no sampling frame exists or where there is a need for speed, non-random sampling methods such as quota sampling and snowball sampling can be used.

Panels may be used to track people's opinions and behaviour over a period of time.

The problems of non-response and deciding on sample size are also discussed.

Introduction

This chapter is about the correct way to take samples of people to be studied. If you do this you will get a sample which can reasonably be regarded as representative of the population from which it has come.

Is the sample representative?

Suppose you want to record what patients on a high protein diet eat when in hospital. You chose to study patients on this diet who are admitted to your hospital in one month. These few patients constitute a sample. Are these patients admitted in a particular month representative of patients admitted throughout the year? Are the patients on a high protein diet admitted to your hospital representative of patients on a high protein diet admitted to hospitals in general?

How can we possibly check whether they are representative? At least we can ask is the food provided in the month we chose to study 'typical' of the food provided in the hospital throughout the year and are the patients admitted in that month typical of patients admitted throughout the year? Similarly we can ask if the food provided in our hospital is 'typical' of that provided in other hospitals and if the criteria for putting someone on a high protein diet are the same in our hospital as elsewhere.

Usually we try to choose a sample in such a way that it will be representative of some larger group. The relationship between populations and samples is shown schematically in Box 7.1. Whenever we have a sample we have to ask is it representative of some larger group?

Box 7.1

Populations and samples

	Example 1	Example 2
Target Population The group to which you wish your findings to be applicable	Patients on a high protein diet	Elderly people living alone
Study Population The group from which you will take a sample to study	Patients on a high protein diet in your hospital	Elderly people living alone in your District and known to one of the statutory services
Study Sample The group you choose to be in the study	Patients on a high protein diet in your hospital during the month of 'fieldwork' of the study	A sample of elderly people living alone in your District and known to one of the statutory services

---

The target population

The group we really wish to study is called the target population. In our previous example this would be all patients on a high protein diet. Other examples of a target population could be all elderly people living alone or all nurses in the West Midlands or all vegetarians in Birmingham. Usually the target population is impossibly difficult to approach directly. You do not know who they are and you have no possible way of finding out. So the target population remains no more than a theoretical concept.

The study population

The first step in the sampling process is defining the study population. The study population is a small but identifiable part of the target population. Examples of possible study populations are all patients in your hospital, all elderly people living alone who are known to the social services, all nurses on the health authority pay roll, all students in hall who have asked for vegetarian meals, all nursing mothers in the district or all children attending local schools.

A 'population' (when a statistician uses the word) need not necessarily be defined in terms of people. A 'population' can just as well be a group of hospitals, wards, schools or old people's homes as the people in them, and how it is defined will depend on the purposes of a study. For example, if you want to compare catering in different hospitals, then hospitals would be the appropriate population, and a list of hospitals would be needed from which to draw a sample. Alternatively, if the purpose is to find out what people think of the catering in your hospital, patients and staff would constitute the appropriate population, and we would need lists of patients and staff.

Different ways of sampling

There are many ways of choosing a sample to represent a population (Table 7.1). We shall spend most time explaining 'Random sampling' methods (confusingly the method is not at all haphazard, as is suggested by its name). A formal definition of random sampling is given in Box 7.2.

There are other methods of sampling which are non-random. 'Quota sampling' is a method much used in market research and 'Snowball sampling' is sometimes used in clinical studies. 'Purposive sampling' is a method of sampling generally used when a representative sample is not wanted.

Table 7.1   Methods of sampling

Random Sampling
   Quasi Random Sampling (Systematic)
   Simple Random Sampling
   Stratified Random Sampling
   Multi-Stage Random Sampling

Non-Random Sampling
   Quota Sampling
   Snowball Sampling
   Purposive Sampling

Box 7.2

Definition of random sample

A Random Sample is one in which every element in the population (sampling frame) has a known, or calculable, and non-zero chance of being included in the sample.

There are three points worth making about this definition.
1   It does *not* say that every element must have an *equal* chance of being included.
2   Every element must have *some* chance of being included (otherwise it would be like missing them off the frame altogether).
3   For samples where the chance of inclusion is not the same for everyone, provided we know (or can calculate) for each what the chance was, then we can use this information to make proper estimates of overall averages.

Simple Random Sample
A Simple Random Sample is one in which every element has an *equal* chance of being included in the sample and every combination of elements has an *equal* chance of being included in the sample.

Box 7.3

Sampling frames

Definition

A frame is a listing of sampling units or elements of the population which we wish to sample.

A frame is perfect if it contains a complete listing of every element in the population: and if every element is included only once.

Possible problems

1 Incomplete coverage (doesn't include every element in the population)
2 Over-coverage (includes elements who/which should not be on the list)
3 Duplication (includes the same element more than once)
4 Clustering (several elements appear at the same place on the frame)

Example 1 – Current in-patients in your hospital

Problems

The patient list is updated in the evening. If the survey is done in the afternoon, patients discharged in the morning will still be on the list.
The frame includes people who should no longer be on it.

Example 2 – Diabetic patients on a list for regular review

Problems

People with diabetes may have moved into the area and *ought* to be called for regular review, but because they have no yet made any contact with the diabetic clinic they are not on the list.
The frame excludes people who should be on it.

Sampling Frame

The first thing you need in order to be able to do random sampling is a list of all the people (or clients) in your study population. This is called a Sampling Frame and is described in Box 7.3. If at all possible you should try to use an existing frame, rather than creating your own. Making up your own frame to suit your specific needs may sound ideal, but you will find that it is very time-consuming. Imagine trying to list every current in-patient in a large hospital independently of the existing admissions list. Even then the frame you have so laboriously created is quite likely to be no more accurate (for the kind of reasons outlined in

Box 7.3) than an existing frame. You should be prepared to compromise on the definition of the study population so that you can use a readily available frame. If you insist on making your own frame recognise that it may involve a lot of extra work.

Simple Random Sampling

Suppose we want to draw a sample of 60 from a population of 600 people. Purists might suggest a method known as Simple Random Sampling. This could be done by writing everyone's name on pieces of paper, putting them into a top hat or tombola, mixing them up and picking out 60. Alternatively we could give everyone a number and pick numbers by using random number tables. Box 7.4 explains how to use random number tables.

Quasi-Random Sampling

Simple random sampling from large populations can be very time consuming and there is an easier way of sampling which is known as Quasi-Random Sampling (Systematic Sampling). This works well provided that the arrangement of the list from which the sample is taken is more or less random with respect to the subject under study. Box 7.5 explains how to do Quasi-Random Sampling.

Quasi-Random Sampling may not work well if the list from which you are sampling is arranged in a systematic or periodic way. Very often lists used for sampling frames are arranged in some ordered way (for example the electoral register is listed in street-number order and an admission list might be in order of admission). List of names arranged in alphabetical order can be used for Quasi-Random Sampling. There are not many personal characteristics linked with the initial letter of surnames, and so sampling from an alphabetic list is likely to be unbiased.

Should you use Quasi-Random Sampling or Simple Random Sampling?

One of the differences between Quasi-Random Sampling and Simple Random Sampling should be obvious. With Quasi-Random Sampling once the random starting point is chosen, the whole sample is fixed. It is not possible, for example, to have the 7th person, the 8th person, the 13th and the 34th in the sample together. With Simple Random Sampling this and all other combinations are possible. Simple Random Sampling has the advantage that it avoids the possible problems which could arise with Quasi-Random Sampling with a systematic or periodic list. Despite the theoretical advantages of Simple Random Sampling over Quasi-Random Sampling, the latter is often used because it is easier to do.

96

Box 7.4

Using random number tables

Random number tables can be found in any standard statistics book or book of mathematical tables.

They look like this:

```
77861  91440  93957  76559  13467  70457  26755  30414  96295  39783
22744  29767  64145  85231  71001  75695  98314  85814  66591  30238
21152  51485  39643  27842  48914  87457  43403  66086  28776  04838
47093  02311  16002  83145  96630  93986  05451  99244  19640  55854
```

The numbers have been specially produced so that there is no pattern for any single digit or combination of digits.

To use the tables to draw a random sample from a sampling frame of 600.
Step 1. Take any block of digits in the table
Step 2. Take the next block of digits to the left
Step 3. Look at the first 3 digits (because 600 has 3 digits)
Step 4a. If the number is 000 or greater than 600 or if the number has already been selected discard the number and go to step 2.
Step 4b. Otherwise select that name from the sampling frame (i.e. if number is 123 take the 123rd name from the sampling frame).

Repeat steps 2 to 4 until you have selected as many as you want in your sample.

The digits are usually printed in blocks so that it is convenient to pick the next block each time but it would not matter if you took any number of digits.

In step 2 you could take the next right, next up, next down etc. It does not matter.

One feature that both Quasi-Random Sampling and Simple Random Sampling have in common is that every individual in the population (on the frame) has an equal chance of being included. There are some random sampling schemes (see Box 7.2) in which different individuals have different but known chances of being included.

Adequate representation of sub-groups

Why, you might ask, would you ever want to take a sample where people have

Box 7.5

Quasi-Random Sampling

Suppose that there are 600 people in the population from which we wish to sample (sampling frame). We want 60 people in our sample.

Step 1 – Finding the sampling interval
The sampling interval is obtained by dividing the size of the population by the desired sample size 600/60 = 10.

We therefore want to sample every 10th person.

Step 2 – Where to start sampling
We could sample the 1st, 11th, 21st, 31st . . . up to the 591st
or the 2nd, 12th, 22nd, 32nd . . . up to the 592nd
and so on.

The first sample should be equal to or less than the sampling interval (i.e. from the first to the tenth) but which of these should we choose? The starting sample should be randomly selected and this is most easily done by using random number tables (see Box 6.4).

Problems with Quasi-Random Sampling in relation to the listing of the frame

1. Systematic list
Suppose hospital patients are listed in order of length of stay (LOS) with the shortest at the top. Any Quasi-Random sample is likely to be biased in terms of LOS. A starting number less than half the sampling interval will underestimate the true average LOS and will bias any measurement associated with LOS, e.g. severity of condition, appreciation (?) of hospital food etc. Conversely a starting number greater than half the sampling interval will over-estimate LOS and bias other measurements accordingly.

2. Periodic list
Suppose people (adults) on a sampling frame are listed in household order, with 'head of the household' first. Such a person is more likely to be male than female. Suppose the population consists mostly of 2-person households. If the sampling interval is an even number, the final sample is likely to consist mostly of men (if the starting number is odd) or of women (if the starting number is even). Knowledge, attitudes etc., are then likely to be biased towards those of whichever sex predominates in the sample.

Despite these theoretical problems Quasi-Random Sampling works well in most situations.

unequal chances of being included? Suppose you want to conduct an opinion survey of hospital food. Vegetarians may well have different opinions of their food from other patients. Certainly, their opinions will be about a different range of foods. Suppose there are only twenty vegetarians in your 600-bed hospital at the time of the survey. If you take a Simple Random Sample by picking the names of sixty patients (all you can afford the time to question) out of a hat, you may well miss all these vegetarians. (The chance of doing this is nearly 1 in 5.) More likely, you might find that your sample only includes one or two vegetarians, which is rather too few to obtain a reliable spectrum of opinion.

To ensure that you have an adequate number of vegetarians (ten is probably a minimum) you would need to over-sample the vegetarians. If the total sample number had to be kept to sixty you would then have to under-sample the non-vegetarians. When presenting overall averages, of course, both the vegetarians and other responses would have to be adjusted to allow for their relative over- and under-representation in the final sample.

Quasi-Random Sampling, Simple Random Sampling and any other method where all members of the population have an equal chance of being included in

---

Box 7.6

Stratified sampling

Definition
All elements of a sampling frame must first be classified in advance by various characteristics relevant to the subject of enquiry. There may be only one of these characteristics (e.g. sex) or there may be several, interlocking with each other (e.g. age and sex, ethnicity). Each sub-group or stratum defined according to a particular combination of characteristics, can then be regarded as a mini-sampling frame in its own right. Sampling occurs within each stratum in accordance with whatever sampling fraction is desired.

Advantages
Stratified sampling ensures that all relevant sub-groups are represented adequately in the final sample. One (statistical) consequence of stratification is reducing the variability of the sample in comparison with other forms of sampling.

Disadvantages
It is necessary to know the relevant characteristics of all members of the sampling frame *before* beginning to sample. This may be difficult, awkward or simply impossible to find out.

the sample all suffer from this important drawback. Small but important groups
may by chance be under sampled. Even if these groups are not undersampled the
sample may still contain too few in that group for worthwhile analysis. The
resolution of this problem is to identify relevant sub-groups in advance, and
make sure they are represented in adequate numbers in the final sample. This
procedure is called Stratified Random Sampling.

Stratified (Random) Sampling

Stratified sampling has a gut appeal because it seems to go a fair way towards
ensuring 'representativeness' of the sample *vis-a-vis* the population. The
different sub-groups within the sampling frame are identified and listed
separately (e.g. Asian men, Asian women, White men, White women). These
separate lists are called strata. A random sample is then drawn separately from
each stratum. Box 7.6 explains how stratified sampling is done.

Post-stratification

Often the relevant information for identifying the sub-groups in the population
(creating the strata) needed for Stratified Random Sampling may not be

available. How then, to proceed? Are we forced back to one of the other two methods described earlier? Not entirely. Although information may not be available in advance about each individual, it is possible that an overall population profile (by age and sex, for example) will be available. If this is so, we can use a procedure known as post-stratification (Box 7.7) to obtain a better estimate of the overall population value.

Another method known as Quota Sampling also depends on the availability of exactly the same kind of information about the population as is necessary for post-stratification. However, the way it works and the underlying theory are completely different from Random Sampling with post-stratification. Quota Sampling is discussed later in this chapter.

Multi-Stage Sampling

All the methods presented so far, Simple Random Sampling, Quasi-Random Sampling and Stratified Sampling require full listings of the sampling frame. In some circumstances such as sampling diets of schoolchildren this may be very difficult to obtain. Each school will have a list of its own children, but a list of all children from all schools may not be available. Similarly, each hospital will have a list of current in-patients, but no overall list of all patients in all hospitals will be kept. One approach would simply be to aggregate the various lists and to sample from this combined list. Alternatively each unit could be regarded as its own stratum and sampling be done directly within each.

Often, however, it is impracticable to think of visiting every school in order to study only five or six children. It would be far more efficient to study thirty in a fewer number of schools. This leads us into a final form of random sampling, often called Multi-Stage Sampling or Cluster Sampling.

In the first stage a sampling frame is drawn up consisting of units such as schools or hospitals or towns. A sample of these units is then taken. Each unit included in the first stage sample then becomes a separate sampling frame for the second stage in which a sample is taken from all the children attending each school or from all the patients attending each hospital. Multi-Stage Sampling is explained further in Box 7.8. It is the method used in most national surveys.

The reason for Random Sampling

The methods outlined above constitute a very quick skim through the main varieties of Random Sampling. Any single random sample drawn on one occasion will not necessarily be 'representative'. However, the importance of the random sampling method is that, on the average, it will guarantee to give a 'representative' sample. No other sampling method offers that guarantee.

Box 7.8

Multi-stage sampling

Clusters, or groups, of individuals exist, e.g. schools (pupils), hospitals (patients), etc. For practical reasons (usually) it is not possible to sample every school or hospital. To begin with, a *sample* of schools/hospitals is taken. If everyone within the chosen schools/hospitals is studied, this is known as *Cluster Sampling*; if a sample of people within the selected schools/hospitals is chosen, this is known as *Multi-Stage Sampling*. The latter is more usual.

NOTE There are two main approaches to Multi-Stage Sampling; they are alternatives and must not be mixed.

1.1 Choose the original sampling units with equal probability, i.e. a small school has the same chance of inclusion as a large school.

1.2 From the list of individuals in each selected unit, choose a constant *proportion*, e.g. 10% of a school of 1000 pupils would give you 100 pupils, whereas 10% of a school of 300 pupils would give you 30 pupils.

2.1 Choose the original sampling units with probability proportional to size, i.e. a school of 1000 pupils would have five times the chance of being included compared with a school of 200 pupils.

2.2 From the list of individuals in each selected unit, choose a constant *number* (e.g. 50) from each unit.

Either of these methods will result in an *equal probability of selection* for every individual on the sampling frame, thus simplifying the calculation of overall averages, etc.

The examples could be extended to embrace three-stage sampling (e.g. hospitals – wards – patients, or schools – classes – pupils) if desired.

Advantages
Multi-Stage Sampling is practically easier than beginning with a large list of everyone in the population. Only at the last stage are lists of individuals required. Fieldwork is necessarily concentrated geographically, and thus easier and cheaper to carry out.

Disadvantages
Missing out a whole cluster (as the method inevitably does) is a bit like missing out whole strata from a sampling process. Whereas stratification usually *increases* the precision of estimates of averages, etc. multi-stage sampling makes the precision *worse*.

Non-Random Sampling

If random sampling is the only method which can guarantee on the average to give a representative sample, why are any non-random sampling methods used at all? Some reasons are clear. Where no sampling frame exists, and none can be created, then some form of non-random sampling is necessary. Other reasons are slightly less obvious. Random Sampling, because it selects specified individuals (and does not allow substitutes) usually turns out to be several times more expensive per completed interview than a non-random method such as quota sampling.

Quota Sampling

Quota Sampling is very widely used in market research and opinion surveys, and certainly has a place in that kind of work. Experience has shown that this method gives estimates of characteristics such as purchasing habits or voting intentions which are sufficiently reliable to be useful. Quota Sampling will not necessarily prove as reliable for studying other characteristics such as health or eating habits.

The essential requirement for Quota Sampling is a 'target population profile', a description of the population in terms of factors such as age, sex and/or whatever else the researcher may feel are important to the subject under study. These factors can be likened to strata used in random sampling. Much information may be available from census data even down to local authority (county/metropolitan borough) level.

Usually we are interested in more than one characteristic of the population, for example age and sex. The number of subjects to be included in each age/sex, etc. category is then set so that the proportions in the quota sample can be related to that in the population from which the sample was taken.

Quota Sampling is most often used in surveys based on interviewing rather than surveys using postal questionnaires. Interviewers go and knock on doors, or stop people in the street, conducting interviews with people who 'fit' one of the available spaces in their quota scheme. There is an obvious difference between this approach and random sampling. In Quota Sampling the interviewers themselves decide both who to approach and whether or not they fit. In random sampling specific, named individuals have to be contacted, and an interviewer has no influence on who is sampled.

Of course, the operational simplicity of Quota Sampling has its drawbacks. Certain kinds of people tend to be under-represented in the final sample (e.g. those who don't go city-centre shopping on Saturdays) and if this characteristic is associated with any of the topics under study, bias of some extent is inevitable. The lack of a sampling frame makes it technically impossible to make reliable assessments of the population you are trying to study and it is never quite clear just who or what the final sample does represent. A summary of the pros and cons of Quota Sampling is given in Box 7.9.

Quota Sampling is sometimes claimed not to suffer the problem of non-response (discussed later in this chapter) because it does not identify specific individuals who have to be included. In fact, the problem is simply disguised. Understandably, poorly trained and supervised interviewers are likely to approach only those people whom they think might answer; and even if a person refuses, the relevant quota can be completed simply by approaching another person (and, if necessary, another) who appears to fit.

Box 7.9

Advantages and disadvantages of Quota Sampling

Advantages	*Disadvantages*
Doesn't require a sampling frame	May be biased in its composition
Quick	Cannot make proper statistical
Cheap	estimates
Requires no knowledge *a priori* of characteristics of individuals	Control of fieldwork difficult
No 'non-response' (but see text)	

Snowball Sampling

Snowball Sampling is used in circumstances where it is impossible to identify a study population because no list or convenient grouping of people exists or can be created. Such might be the case with, for example, a rare medical condition or disability, where the two or three people known to a specialist in this hospital happen to know a couple of others who go to another hospital, who also know others and so on. Again, the notion of a target population is clear, but the study population is well-nigh impossible to define, and the study sample becomes simply that which you can get hold of by asking someone already in the study if they know anyone else with the same condition.

Purposive Sampling

All the sampling methods discussed so far have attempted to obtain a representative sample. Purposive Sampling is different in that it is often deliberately intended to select a non-representative sample. The way we choose fruit in the supermarket is an example of purposive sampling. We choose fruit carefully, so that it is free of blemishes and is neither under- or over-ripe. The population (of fruit) is laid out before us and we choose what we want and what we think is the best. In no sense is the aim to obtain an 'average' or representative sample of fruits. We want the best available.

Of course it is possible to change the element of judgement such that the declared aim is to obtain a representative sample as you might when taking sweets from a 'pick and mix' selection. This might make sense when selecting patients for a preliminary study of their views on catering.

However, your judgement of what is a representative group of patients is likely to be very different from someone else's. The elements of judgement involved provide no guarantee of agreement on what or who is representative.

A slightly different use of Purposive Sampling is when you want to look at the range of opinions in a study population. You will then select patients to make sure they included extreme views as well as moderate views. Purposive Sampling is not often used by survey workers though it may be suitable for pilot studies or in-depth studies where you intend to study very small numbers.

Panels

Panels are not a method of sampling as such, rather they are a particular way of using a sample obtained through any one of the rigorous (or not so rigorous) methods outlined above. One purpose of having a panel is to obtain information about how people's habits and/or opinions change over time (longitudinal information).

We might for example use a panel to study trends in food buying and consumption patterns. If such information is obtained about one group of individuals this year and another group next year, we cannot be sure whether any differences observed are because (i) the time is different, (ii) the individuals are different, (iii) both of these, or (iv) some other reason(s). With a panel of people who will respond to questions on several occasions over time, we can at least be sure that the people are the same and that reasons for any changes observed must lie elsewhere.

Selecting a panel

In principle any of the various sampling procedures already described could be used to select a panel. However the nature of the activity people are being invited to join must be explained even more carefully than usual to potential participants. It is unrealistic, for example, to expect to be able to acquire a suitably committed panel from a series of street-corner quota sample interviews. Random sampling, whilst theoretically superior as a sampling method, has few advantages when choosing a panel.

Here it is helpful to reconsider what we might hope to obtain from a panel. The twin (and sometimes conflicting) aims of validity and generalisability must be considered. Generalisability means that we want to be able to assert that the results from our sample can be regarded as representative of the population. Validity, on the other hand, is concerned with the 'internal' respectability of the sample results *per se*. Validity can be obtained, often at the expense of generalisability, by careful selection of participants to join a panel. If there is a large drop-out rate over time, the results will have little validity as far as the original sample is concerned (though they may be entirely valid for those individuals who stayed the course) and no generalisability. In the context of panel surveys, where people may need persuading to take part over an extended period of time, it is more important that the results obtained should be valid for the participating individuals than that they should be generalisable.

Problems with panels

Some of the problems with panels have already been mentioned. Representativeness is the first of these. Panel members may represent no one other than those who could be persuaded to take part. Dropping out is another problem. If membership of a panel is extended over a long period of time, members may be lost from the panel through moving house, non-cooperation through weariness or boredom and death. A quite different problem is that of acclimatisation. Simply being on the panel, and answering a series of questions about food and eating changes the way you behave, your food purchase and eating patterns, or simply your attitudes to and knowledge about the subject of study.

Non-response

Non-response should be regarded as a problem in all sampling schemes because the people who do not respond have already shown themselves in one respect (responding) to be unlike those who do. They may therefore be dissimilar in other matters relevant to the subject of study. There are many kinds of non-response, ranging from those who were missed off the sampling frame (and therefore never had a chance of responding) to those who were never in when an interviewer called, those who couldn't understand the questions and those who refused point-blank to answer or simply throw away a postal questionnaire. Different types of non-response may nevertheless provide different amounts of information about the individual concerned. For example, face-to-face refusal should at least provide some idea of the age, sex and ethnicity of the non-responder whereas none of this information may be known for a non-responder to a postal questionnaire.

So what can be done about non-response in random sampling? Repeat calls or repeat postal questionnaires are obvious and worthwhile approaches, though the cost of sending interviewers back to the same address several times can rapidly blow the budget. For both types of questionnaire there is no substitute for a carefully worded introduction, or covering letter. This should engage the interest and attention of the potential subject without putting them off because too much appears to be asked of them. Comparing characteristics of those who respond first time and those who only respond after a reminder or those who respond quickly and those who respond after a delay may reveal differences. This sort of information may enable you to make some estimate of the likely characteristics of the non-responders. Non-responders may resemble the slow or reluctant responders more closely than they resemble the quick responders.

One approach is to use substitutes but this is not a universal panacea. If your random sample indicates you should select this person (and they never seem to be in, or don't reply to your postal questionnaire) selecting the next person off the sampling frame is (a) biased (because that person has had more than a normal chance of being included) and (b) like quota sampling, simply hides the fact and extent of non-response. It has to be recognised that poor response rates may be a reflection of poor research (including questionnaire) design. A thirty percent response rate from an approach to 1000 people is less representative of the target population than a ninety percent response rate from 200 people.

Sample size

'How big a sample size do I need?' is probably the commonest question asked of a statistician. There isn't a simple answer.

In most circumstances the limiting factor will be the resources of the research worker, money, time, equipment and so on. For obvious practical reasons the numbers of people who can be cajoled into doing a month-long weighed intake survey are fewer than those who can be questioned as to their opinions of fast food products.

If sample size has been fixed by practical constraints then the question becomes 'what can I reasonably expect to discover with a sample of this size?'. It may become clear that you cannot achieve your original aim with the sample size proposed. In this case you must either change your aim to one which you can achieve with your sample size or you must go off and find more resources so that you can increase your sample size.

Statistical methods are needed to show what you can reasonably hope to do with a given sample size. They can answer questions such as 'How accurately can I estimate the mean fat intake in this group?' or 'How accurately can I estimate the proportion of people who drink skim milk in that group?' or 'If there is a difference between this group and that group what is the smallest difference I could expect to detect?'. Questions such as these are relevant to almost every type of survey enquiry, and the researcher should ensure that they are asked

Box 7.10

How big a sample 1?

Example 1 – A descriptive study of frequency
Suppose that studies elsewhere suggest that about 60% of men 'usually' eat wholemeal bread. You would like to know whether the proportion in your district is more than, less than, or much the same as, this 60%. How many people do you need to ask? Because of taking a sample, we can only be accurate to within certain limits – say plus or minus 5% of the true value (or ±10%, or ±3% and so on – the choice is yours). Furthermore, we can only achieve that accuracy with a certain degree of confidence – 95% is common, but 90% and 99% are also used. In the end, we can make statements of the following kind: we are 95% certain of estimating the true population proportion to within ±7%, and to do this we need a sample size of N.

Information needed to calculate the required sample size (an example)
'Guesstimate' of what the population proportion might be	p	60%
'Accuracy factor' – estimate p to within ±5%	a	5%
'Confidence factor' – how sure do we want to be		95%

Sample sizes required for different population proportions, accuracy factors and confidence factors.

'Guesstimate' of population proportion	Confidence factor					
	95%			99%		
	Accuracy factor			Accuracy factor		
	10%	5%	3%	10%	5%	3%
50%	97	385	1068	167	666	1849
60%	93	369	1025	160	640	1776
75%	73	289	801	125	500	1387
90%	35	139	385	60	240	666

For proportions less than 50%, look up 100% minus population percent (e.g. for 25%, look up $100 - 25 = 75\%$).
The formula for calculating the required sample size N is:
$$N = \frac{p(100-p)\,t^2}{a^2}$$
Where p = 'guesstimate' of the population proportion
    a = the accuracy factor
    t = a measurement corresponding to the confidence factor.
        t is the 'standard normal deviate' and can be looked up in statistical tables. Its precise value depends on the sample size but the most commonly used values used are given below:

Confidence factor	90%	95%	99%
t-value	1.65	1.96	2.58

Box 7.11

How big a sample 2?

Example 2 – A descriptive study of a mean
We want to find out the mean daily consumption of iron by pregnant mothers in our district. Carrying out a survey is the obvious way to proceed – how big a sample do we need?

As with the previous example (Box 7.10) we have to decide on the 'accuracy factor' (let this be 1mg/day) and the 'confidence factor' (let this be 95%). That is, we want to be 95% certain of estimating the mean in the population to within ±1mg/day of its true value.

We need one extra piece of information, an estimate of the population standard deviation (SD) (see Box 16.4). Suppose we know from other surveys that this is about 4mg/day.

Information needed to calculate the required sample size:

'Guesstimate' of what the population SD might be	SD	4mg/day
Accuracy factor – estimate to within 1mg/day	a	1mg/day
Accuracy factor as fraction of SD	a/SD	0.25
Confidence factor – how sure do we want to be		95%

Sample sizes for different accuracy factors (as fraction of SD) and confidence factors

	Confidence factor							
	95%				99%			
	Accuracy factor as fraction of SD				Accuracy factor as fraction of SD			
	0.5	0.25	0.1	0.005	0.5	0.25	0.1	0.005
Required sample size	16	62	385	1537	27	107	666	2663

The formula for calculating required sample size is:

$$N = \left(\frac{t\,SD}{a}\right)^2$$

Where t is measurement corresponding to the confidence factor: see Box 7.10.

These calculations assume that the measurement has a Gaussian distribution in the population.

Box 7.12

How big a sample 3?

Example 3 – Analytical study of differences in proportions
We want to ascertain the effect of a healthy eating campaign in the district and in particular to find out whether the true proportion of adults eating fresh fruit most days has changed. We are going to do this by taking a sample before the campaign and then another sample afterwards. Assuming the two samples will be of equal size how many adults should we have in each sample?

We need to know the proportion of regular fruit eaters in the district before the campaign and to state the smallest difference that we would be interested in knowing about (e.g. a 1% difference would be trivial, a 5% difference might be of interest and a 10% difference definitely would). This smallest difference of interest is rather like, but not exactly the same, as the accuracy factor in Boxes 7.10 and 7.11.

The confidence factor has to be stated again but in this case we also need to state a power factor – an indication of how often we might fail to find a difference when one really did exist. In a 'powerful test' the power factor might be as high as 95% (a failure rate of 5%) but more usually it is set at 90% or 80%.

Information needed to calculate the required sample sizes:

'Guesstimate' of initial proportion	p_1	40%
Difference to be detected	D	+ 10%
Confidence factor		95%
Power factor		80%

This means you have an 80% chance of finding a 10% change in the proportion of adults who are regular fruit eaters when such a difference exists and a 5% chance of finding such a difference when it does not really exist.

Sample sizes needed to detect specified size differences with 80% power.

	Confidence factor							
	95%				99%			
% Initial	Size of change				Size of change			
proportion	− 20	− 10	+ 10	+ 20	− 20	− 10	+ 10	+ 20
10	–	–	156	41	–	–	229	60
30	74	317	336	84	113	476	499	125
50	95	389	389	95	143	581	581	143
60	94	378	369	89	140	564	552	134
80	67	262	233	52	99	358	353	80

Continued opposite

The formula for calculating sample size is:

$$N = \left(\frac{z_1 \sqrt{2p_1(100-p_1)} + z_2 \sqrt{p_1(100-p_1) + p_2(100-p_2)}}{D} \right)^2$$

Where $p_2 = p_1 + D$

Values for z_1	95%	1.96	99%	2.58		
z_2	80%	0.84	90%	1.28	95%	1.65

With all sample size calculations if you are unsure about what you need to do, whether you need to do it or how to do it CONSULT A STATISTICIAN BEFORE YOU START.

before the work is begun rather than after. (Well, how many subjects should I have studied, then?)

In a book such as this, detailed discussion of the methods of calculating sample size requirements for different studies is not appropriate, but some general principles can at least be outlined. Some examples of sample size calculation are given in Boxes 7.10, 7.11 and 7.12.

Roughly speaking, we can divide studies into two kinds, descriptive and analytical.

Descriptive studies will largely be concerned with describing food consumption patterns, cholesterol levels and so on in samples of individuals. For these studies, the appropriate question is 'How accurately can I estimate the sample mean with a given sample size?' or 'How accurately can I estimate the proportions in different categories?'. The answer to these questions will depend partly on the sample size and partly on the distribution of the characteristics within the study population. Estimates of the mean are less accurate if there is a wide range of values in the population.

Analytical studies tend to concentrate on identifying differences between groups, and for these, the second type of question will be more suitable: 'How big a sample do I need to show a difference between groups?'. The answer to this question depends on the distribution of the characteristic in the groups and the size of the difference between them. Small differences are more difficult to demonstrate than larger differences and any difference is harder to demonstrate when there is wide variation within the groups.

In both instances, it is recommended that the issue be brought to, and discussed with, a statistician at the nearest polytechnic or university before starting or the project may be found to be full of holes just as it is launched.

Further reading

Lemeshow S., Hosmer D. W., Klar J. and Lwanga S. K. (1990)
   Adequacy of sample size in health studies. WHO, Wiley, Chichester.

8 · Process evaluation – describing what was done

by Neil J. G. Field

Summary

Process evaluation involves describing the activities in a promotion of healthier eating. Detailed study of these activities can throw light on how the promotion is working and suggest ways in which it could be made more effective. It can be used as a progress-chasing device so that any problems can be identified and set right quickly.

Four examples are given to illustrate the use of process evaluation. These examples are (1) a healthy eating leaflet (2) a healthy eating display (3) a training event for cooks and (4) a healthy eating talk/lecture.

'Outcome' and 'Process' – different types of evaluation

The word 'outcome' is used to describe the final results of our activities while the word 'process' describes the activities themselves. Outcome evaluation seeks to quantify the effectiveness of our activities by looking at their outcomes. Process evaluation is best understood as 'describing' the activity which was undertaken. It is needed in addition to the outcome evaluation in order to understand the effectiveness of the programme or intervention and gain insights on how the success was achieved or missed.

An example will illustrate the difference between outcome and process evaluation. Consider a promotion of healthier food purchase intended to influence people to buy more wholemeal loaves and fresh fruit. The outcome evaluation would ask how many extra wholemeal loaves and how much more fresh fruit have been sold during the promotion and attempt to assess whether this change was caused by the promotion.

The process evaluation would ask questions such as: how were the wholemeal loaves and fresh fruit promoted? Were they offered at a specially low cash price or were people given coupons which they could exchange for these products? Was there a national or local advertising campaign? Were they offered in a new packaging and how prominently were they displayed at the point of sale?

The differences between summative evaluation and formative evaluation were described in Chapter 1. Note that a summative evaluation is chiefly an outcome evaluation while formative evaluations tend to be chiefly process evaluations.

Why describe activities?

When a promotions programme or planned intervention is undertaken we ought to evaluate how it went and seek to understand the reasons for the success or failure. Unless we look carefully at the ways that it was undertaken and the activities that went into it we cannot guess why the promotion was a success or failure. It is all very interesting to know that there was a 12% increase in sales over two months but unless we also know what was done to produce this result we cannot learn from our experience or implement the intervention elsewhere.

Studying and describing activities have the important advantage of giving continued feedback while the promotion is going on. We can thus quickly identify the strengths and weaknesses of the programme while it is running and make necessary modifications before many resources have been wasted. It also serves as a useful way of chasing progress and provides information to reassure the funding source. This has particular importance with long term intervention programmes.

We will now look at some examples of how studying process can be useful in a number of promotional and intervention programmes.

The problem of linking process and outcome

This chapter deals predominantly with the question 'What was done?' (process evaluation). Other chapters deal with the question 'Did anything change?'. There is however a third and very important question 'Was the change observed caused by whatever was done?' The first two questions have to be answered before we can tackle this third and most difficult question.

Often (as in this chapter) the activities described are simply assumed to be responsible for any change observed. This is most likely to be true with small-scale short-term activity and least likely to be true with large long-term programmes. In complex programmes lasting months or years there are many things other than your activities which could cause change and you cannot assume that you are responsible for any change observed. Methods for helping you decide the cause of change are described in Chapter 4.

Example 1 – A leaflet on healthy eating

It has been decided to produce in conjunction with a local retailer a leaflet extolling the benefits of eating breads with a higher fibre content. Before producing the leaflet, work was done to show that information on this topic was needed and to identify who it was that needed the information. The leaflet was then designed and produced to supply this information and to be suitable for the identified target group. The outcome evaluation could be one or both of:

114

i   interviewing shoppers on knowledge, attitude and behaviour before and after having read the leaflet.

ii   measuring the change in sales of higher fibre breads and how these may have been affected by the distribution of the leaflet.

The description of process (activity) could well include the following:

i   How many leaflets were printed and how much did it cost to produce them?

ii   How were they distributed? Where and how were they displayed? Did shoppers have to pick them up themselves or were the leaflets given to them?

iii   How were the methods and outlets for leaflet distribution chosen?

iv   How quickly were the leaflets taken? Were they placed into every shopper's basket?

v   Were the leaflets used as part of other initiatives such as discounting or coupon promotion? Were they used as part of a point of sale promotion and placed close to the foods being promoted?

By looking through this list, which is not exhaustive, we can see how useful this information is in telling us how the leaflet was used. For example if very few people took the leaflet because it was displayed in a way that made people think they had to pay for it, then this could be put right quickly. The leaflet in the store could be placed in other parts of the store to find which position gave maximum uptake. The information gathered will be of interest to those who paid for or commissioned the campaign. Process evaluation will give you an opportunity to discuss your findings with them as you gather the information.

Example 2 – A display on healthy eating

The next example is a display about healthy eating. This might be a choice selection of 'healthier items' in a canteen or food store, a board display encouraging lower fat consumption, or a display presenting planned improvements to school meals by education caterers for use at parent evenings. We can assume that a need for some form of information provision or awareness raising has been identified and that the display has been designed to meet this need.

The outcome evaluation would seek to produce evidence of change in awareness of the issue, knowledge, attitude or behaviour as a result of the display.

115

The process evaluation will, through describing the activities, endeavour to shed some light on how many changes were achieved. For example:

i   Who constructed and organised the display and how long did it take them?

ii   What was the cost of the display?

iii   How was the display used? Was it unattended or were health education or other staff present?

iv   Where was the display sited? What other places could have been used?

v   Did the display attract attention? How many people looked at the display and did they just glance at it or look at it in detail?

vi   Did one part of the display attract more interest or cause more comment than another?

Continuing evaluation of this nature each time the display is used will have the effect of ensuring the best possible use is made of the display. It may help you understand how the changes in knowledge, attitudes or awareness measured in the outcome evaluation were achieved.

Example 3 – A training event for cooks

Cooks may need to change their practices in order to implement healthy eating policies. Staff training is an important aspect of health promotion. Unless people understand the reasons for the changes and how to effect them, then a healthy eating policy will be thwarted by ignorance, apathy or incompetence. Training, like other health promotion activity should be evaluated.

The long-term outcome evaluation should involve improvement of sales or uptake of the 'healthier' items or menus. In the short term, a questionnaire given to the cooks at completion of the training will give some idea as to their immediate impressions as to the usefulness of the training and even whether they have started to put into practice some of what they have learnt.

The process evaluation will seek to answer some of these questions:

i   Who was included in the training event? Why were these people chosen and why were other people not chosen?

ii   Where did the training take place? Was the venue comfortable and conducive to learning?

iii   What were the costs? Who paid them?

iv   How many of the cooks who were invited attended?

v   Who did the training?

vi   What topics were included in the training?

vii   What methods of training were used? Talks, discussion groups, practical demonstrations, videos, films, etc?

viii   Which parts of the event did the trainers feel went well and which parts did they feel went badly?

By comparing the answers to these questions with the cook's impressions of the course we can quickly find out which parts of the training were relevant and acceptable. We can also obtain some clues as to why the training event was a success (or failure). We can use the experience to improve any future training events and to make them more effective.

Example 4 – Talks and lectures on healthy eating

As part of the implementation of a healthy food policy, many types of talks, lectures and presentations have to be made to many different groups of people such as a local authority committee, a group of chief officers, a purchasing department, retailers, students, etc. Before the talk you will have clarified what the talk is intended to achieve, what you hope the audience will learn from the talk and what the speaker hopes to learn from the audience.

The outcome evaluation will, in its simplest form, be: Did they make the desired changes? Sometimes it may be appropriate to ask the group to complete a post-talk questionnaire. For other groups this method may not be acceptable and you would lose all credibility with some audiences (for example senior politicians) if you asked them to complete a questionnaire shortly after your presentation.

The process evaluation should seek answers to these questions:

i   Why was the presentation made to the group?

ii   Who was included in the group and why?

iii   Why was the venue chosen?

iv   What was the content of the presentation?

117

v   How did the 'audience' react to the information, to the way in which it was presented and to the speaker?

vi What follow-up is needed? By the group? By the presenter?

Conclusion

The examples given are not exhaustive and may be inappropriate for your use, but the underlying principles are applicable to all promotions, interventions and training.

Many understand the term evaluation to mean only 'let us look at the outcome of our activity' (outcome evaluation). This chapter has shown that you also have to look closely at the activities undertaken (the process) in order to understand how the outcome was achieved and how the activities can be modified to give an even better result next time. Detailed studies of process provide the basis for more efficient use of health promotion resources and more effective promotion of healthier eating.

9 · Measurement of knowledge of food and nutrition

Summary

Better knowledge is an important part of strategies for promotion of healthier eating. This is true for health promotion based on traditional KAB (Knowledge Attitude Behaviour) models and for health promotion based on empowerment models. Therefore, measurements of knowledge are needed to inform planning of effective health promotion activities and monitoring of its implementation.

The measurement should concentrate on areas of knowledge which are necessary for substantially healthier food choices and should cover the specific areas on which the health promotion was focused.

Open questions can be useful for assessing knowledge in small groups. Closed questions in true-false or multiple choice format are generally more suitable for large scale or postal surveys. All types of question have to be unambiguous, of an appropriate level of difficulty and as little affected as possible by respondent characteristics other than knowledge of healthy eating.

Knowledge and belief

A belief is what someone holds to be true. Whether a belief is classified as knowledge depends on whether it is accepted as true. A belief that one person calls knowledge, may be considered by another person to be merely opinion (perhaps true, perhaps false) and may even be regarded by someone else as dogma (an irrational belief) or myth (a false belief).

In the context of promotion of healthier eating the knowledge that is important is useful information about the healthiness of relevant eating habits and food choices.

Why measure knowledge?

The first reason for measuring knowledge of food and nutrition is the hope that this knowledge affects eating behaviour. To be sure, knowledge by itself is not enough to influence behaviour. In many situations an improvement in knowledge may have little effect. None-the-less in other situations, when attitudes are favourable and opportunities for change exist, better knowledge may have a powerful effect on behaviour. The question of how knowledge and attitudes affect behaviour is discussed further in Chapter 10.

Another reason for measuring knowledge is that it is clearly a necessary condition for informed choice about eating. If someone knows the effect of different foods on their health then they are empowered to choose (or reject) those foods. Someone who knows the nutrient content of foods and understands the principles of healthier eating has much more choice in constructing their diet than someone who only has a list of foods which they believe to be bad for them.

This is not an exam!

It is important to realise, that in the context of health promotion, knowledge measurement is never about identifying 'failures'. This must always be made crystal clear to respondents and measurement of knowledge must not be allowed to resemble 'exams' or 'school tests'. The main purpose is to tell the health promoters about what further information might be needed by the people with whom they work.

Assessment of knowledge is also used in health education to give feedback to the people whose knowledge is being measured. However, instruments which are good for giving feedback to respondents are often not suitable for collecting information for planning or programme evaluation and so it is usually best to do the two things separately.

What ought people to know? – 'know that' and 'know how'

The first step is to decide the points of information which we want people to know. We cannot measure any knowledge until we have decided precisely what it is that we are trying to measure.

In planning health education a baseline survey will be helpful to check how many people already have important points of information, how certain they are about this knowledge and to what extent they use it. After the health education activity, further surveys will show whether the knowledge objectives have been met.

Box 9.1 shows areas of nutrition knowledge as they might be listed in a textbook of nutrition and dietetics. For health promotion we need to organise the knowledge in rather a different way, concentrating on items of information that are practically useful in making food and eating choices. Box 9.2 shows selected areas of knowledge organised to be relevant to health promotion and covers 'know that' information which provides a reason for making healthier choices and 'know how' information which enables people to put the 'know that' information into practice or even to eat healthily without understanding why.

The items of information to be included in a measure of nutritional knowledge will differ for each population. The list that would be appropriate for a group of

Box 9.1

**Areas of knowledge of food and nutrition
(arranged as for textbook)**

1   *Chemical nature of nutrients*
    Starches, sugar, fats, saturated and unsaturated fatty acids, proteins

2   *Physiological function of foods*
    Starch and complex carbohydrates, sugars, proteins, fats
    Vitamins, sodium, potassium, calcium, iron, trace minerals

3   *Dietary causes of disease*
    Total fat and heart disease, saturated fat and heart disease
    Dietary fibre and bowel function, dietary fibre and colon cancer
    Sugar and dental caries
    Vitamin deficiency states

4   *Nutrient content of food*
    High fat and low fat foods, types of fat in foods
    High fibre and low fibre foods
    High protein and low protein foods, high energy and low energy foods
    Sources of vitamins and minerals

5   *Shopping and food preparation techniques*

6   *'Healthy eating rules'*
    Eat less fat
    Eat less saturated fat
    Eat more dietary fibre
    Eat more fruit and vegetables
    Eat breakfast!
    Avoid calories if you are only thirsty

---

dieticians is different from that appropriate for a group of doctors and different again from that appropriate for a group of business people or factory production workers.

You might think that it is unimportant for people to know what the various nutrients are or what they do, so long as they know how to choose and prepare 'healthy meals'. In this case your knowledge measurement would cover only some simple 'healthy eating rules' (basic 'know how'). On the other hand you might have some evidence that it is important that people understand how diet

Box 9.2

Areas of knowledge of healthier eating 1 – Fats in the diet

TOTAL FAT

Know that	*Know how*

Increases risk of heart disease and certain cancers	Lower fat food preparation:
	    Grilling/steaming/boiling as
	        alternatives to frying

Fat rich foods are calorie dense	Trimming visible fat off meat Skinning chickens
Need to reduce total fat intake of adults	Draining fats after cooking mince Fat reduction in recipes

Fat intake of under 5s should not be reduced	Possible exchanges to lower fat:
	    Skimmed/semi-skimmed milk for
	        full fat milk
	    Low fat spread for butter/marge
	    Yoghurt for cream
	    Jacket/boiled potatoes for chips

	Use sparingly to lower fat:
	    Spreads; cheeses; meat products
	    (mince, sausages etc)

POLYUNSATURATED FATS

Polyunsaturated fats different from saturated fats	Need to read labels on spreads to find polyunsaturate content
Do not need to reduce intake of polyunsaturates	Possible exchanges to increase polyunsaturates:
Should not increase intake of polyunsaturates too much	Flora/Vitalite/Other poly rich for butter/other poly low spreads
Polyunsaturates may protect against heart disease	Sunflower/safflower oils etc for 'mixed vegetable'/other poly low oils
Polyunsaturates reduce serum cholesterol	Poly rich fats in cooking for hard fats
Some but not all plant oils are rich sources of polyunsaturates	Fish for beef/sheep/pig meat
Fishes are source of polyunsaturates	

Continued opposite

affects their health so that they can work out their own ways of 'healthy eating'. In this case it would be important to measure their knowledge of 'know that' information as well as of more extensive 'know how' information. 'Know that' information should cover the dietary causes of disease and the physiological actions of nutrients. 'Know how' could cover the nutrient content of foods. Before we can properly design measures of knowledge we have to have information on eating habits. Then we can concentrate on those items of knowledge about food, eating and health on areas which are practically helpful in making food choices.

The measurement of knowledge

Questions for estimating knowledge should have these characteristics:
    Free from ambiguity
    Appropriate level of difficulty (not too easy, not too hard)
    Unaffected by subject characteristics unrelated to knowledge

Type of question – open or closed

Questions intended to measure knowledge can be open or closed. Examples of open ended questions are:

Can you name three foods which contain fibre?

Can you name three things which increase the risk of getting heart disease?

The same knowledge could be explored by questions asked in a closed form.

These foods contain fibre:

Milk	True	False
Apples	True	False
Bread	True	False
Potatoes	True	False

Do these habits increase your risk of getting heart disease?

Smoking	Yes	No
Taking physical exercise	Yes	No
Having high blood pressure	Yes	No
Eating a lot of fatty foods	Yes	No

Open questions to assess knowledge

With individuals or small groups the most effective way of measuring their knowledge may well be open ended questions in an interview or questionnaire. Open ended questions are however difficult to score.

For example the question 'What is dietary fibre?' might attract the following answers:

'The stringy pieces in fruit and vegetables'

'It's bran'

'It's stuff which stops you getting constipated'

'It's the constituents of plant cell walls'

'Fibre is cellulose and hemicellulose'

'Dietary fibre is material of plant origin which is incompletely digested by human alimentary enzymes'

Which (if any) of these answers is completely correct? How do you score the different pieces of information contained in these replies? Each one shows some understanding of the nature of dietary fibre.

This question as it was asked causes problems because it did not make clear to the respondent precisely what information was required. It would have been better to ask initially 'What foods contain a lot of fibre?' and then perhaps 'Are there different sorts of dietary fibre?' and 'What does each do?' Open questions are most useful when they are precise but not leading. When used in interviews, the answer (or lack of answer) to open question can be followed up by prompts such as 'Can you give any other foods which contain fibre?', 'Does it do anything else?' and so on, but always taking care that these prompts do not suggest specific answers.

The open question can give very rich information and so tends to be more suitable for exploring knowledge of more complicated topics. It also tends to be more difficult because the question gives no clue as to the correct answer, unlike the closed question which inevitably provides the correct answer among several incorrect ones. Open questions take more time to process and are more difficult to score. Thus open questions can give very helpful qualitative information but are generally not suited to quantitative assessment of knowledge.

Closed questions to assess knowledge

Most or all questions in a larger survey will almost certainly have to be closed. Questions may be set in true-false or multiple choice formats.

True-false format

Questions need to be clear so that everyone interprets them in the same way. How should one answer questions like 'Semi-skimmed milk contains very little fat – True or False?' or 'Potato is a good source of vitamin C – True or False'. The questions depend on interpretation of the words 'very little' and 'good source'.

The same areas of knowledge are better assessed by questions of the type: 'Semi-skimmed milk contains less fat than whole milk — True or False?' or 'A usual helping of potato contains half the adult daily requirement for vitamin C – True or False'. This avoids the use of vague words describing quantity, though the phrase 'usual helping' could still cause problems.

There is a danger that in trying to avoid ambiguity we make the questions too difficult; for example 'One hundred grammes of boiled new potatoes contains about 15 mg vitamin C – True or False' contains no ambiguity but is testing a very abstruse and practically unimportant area of knowledge.

There is also a danger that in the effort to remove all ambiguity or to make questions more difficult we produce questions which are too complicated. Such questions test ability to understand long words and complex sentences rather than nutritional knowledge.

The wording of statements should be simple and negatives should as far as possible be avoided. For example, the question:

Cholesterol in food is not the most important dietary factor influencing blood cholesterol – True or False

would be much better restated as:

Blood cholesterol comes mostly from cholesterol eaten in food – True or False

or:

High intake of saturated fats in the diet is the main dietary cause of high blood cholesterol — True or False.

False statements should be chosen so that superficial knowledge suggests a wrong answer. Possible questions are:

Butter contains mostly polyunsaturated fats   True or False
Polyunsaturated fats raise blood cholesterol   True or False

Trick questions should not be used to produce likely looking false statements. For example, the question:

The legal limit for blood alcohol in drivers is 80 mg/l – True or False – is a poor question because it is testing the ability to spot a wrong unit (it should be 80 mg/dl) rather than knowledge of the limit.

True-false questions are sometimes arranged in blocks. For example:

Two slices of bread supply more than one tenth of the daily requirement for these vitamins

Vitamin A	True	False
Vitamin B1 (Thiamin)	True	False
Vitamin B2 (Niacin)	True	False
Vitamin D	True	False

Breaking them into short blocks like this improves the appearance and readability of the set of questions.

The number of true-false questions in which 'true' is the correct answer should be roughly the same in a quiz as the number in which 'false' is correct. If most of the correct answers are 'true' then people who have a tendency (response set) to answer 'yes' will score more highly than their knowledge warrants.

True-false items are not easy to write but if care is taken they can give highly valid measures of knowledge. An example of true-false format questions on choosing lower fat foods is given in Box 9.3.

Multiple choice format

In multiple choice questions, there are a stem and several possible answers. The respondent has to select the correct answer or the best answer. As for true-false

Box 9.3

True-false format quiz on fat content of foods

Please indicate whether the following statements are true or false by marking each one with a T or an F.

1 Cottage cheese contains more fat than Edam cheese   (F)

2 Chicken (without the skin) contains more fat than lamb   (F)

3 Boiled potatoes are low in fat   (T)

4 Skimmed milk contains almost as much fat as whole milk   (F)

5 Grilling can reduce the fat content of bacon and sausage   (T)

6 Butter and margarine have the same total fat content   (T)

7 Edam cheese contains less fat than Cheddar cheese   (T)

8 Low fat spread contains less than one quarter the fat of butter   (F)

9 Chips are higher in fat than roast potatoes   (T)

10 Salad cream contains the same amount of fat as mayonnaise   (F)

11 Skinless chicken contains more fat than chicken with skin   (F)

12 Rich fruit cake contains less fat than sponge cake   (F)

13 Skimmed milk contains less fat than semi-skimmed milk   (T)

14 All soft spreads are lower in fat than hard spreads   (F)

15 All nuts contain more fat than raisins   (T)

16 Plain ice-cream wafers contain more fat than digestive biscuits   (F)

Note the Ts and Fs in brackets refer to the correct answers for coding responses. Of course they should not appear on the document presented to a respondent!

questions, the statements need to be unambiguous and written in clear and simple language. It is important that there should be one and only one correct option for each question. For example consider the question item:

Your risk of getting heart disease is increased by eating a diet:
A)   Rich in fibre
B)   Rich in cholesterol
C)   Rich in fat
D)   Low in iron
E)   Low in calcium

This is a bad item because, although C is the best answer, B (and possibly E) are also true.

The possible answers which are wrong (distractors) have to look as though they might be right. In the previous example a diet rich in fibre acts as a 'distractor' because those who have heard that fibre has something to do with risk of heart disease may mistakenly select it as the correct answer.

Care must be taken that clues are not included in the stem as for example in the question:

It has been suggested that average fibre intake should be increased from 20 grammes per day to:
A)   10 grammes per day
B)   15 grammes per day
C)   25 grammes per day
D)   30 grammes per day.

The use of the word increased in the stem makes it obvious that options A and B are wrong.

The possible answers should be presented in some natural order (e.g. alphabetical, numerical, etc.). The position of the correct option should be random throughout the questions. It is no good writing a list of questions in which the first option is always wrong and the middle option is most frequently right.

Checklists for writing true-false and multiple choice questions are given in Box 9.4.

Level of difficulty

It is important that the level of difficulty should be appropriate for the group being studied. A questionnaire which worked well in testing the knowledge of a group of dieticians would probably not work well with a group of shoppers. One

128

Box 9.4

Checklist for closed questions

1   For true-false questions
1   Is each item expressed in clear, simple language?
2   Have negative statements been avoided as far as possible?
3   Have trick questions been removed?
4   Is each item clearly true or false?
5   Are there approximately the same number of true and false items and are they randomly distributed through the quiz?

2   For multiple choice items
1   Has the item been clearly presented?
2   Has the item been written so as to avoid repetition of phrases in each option?
3   Have the responses been arranged in some natural order?
4   Are all the distractors plausible?
5   Have all clues (grammatical, length of answer, etc.) been avoided in the stem statement?
6   Are the correct answers randomly positioned throughout the test?
7   Have negative statements been avoided? If a negative statement is used has the negative been emphasised (underlined or written in capitals)?
8   Have overlapping options been avoided?
9   Is there one and only one correct option for each stem?

3   For all question formats
1   Have the questions been independently reviewed by an expert in the area of knowledge?
2   Has the scoring system been validly constructed?
3   Has the questionnaire been validated?

---

needs a questionnaire where the most knowledgeable members of the group get most (but not all) of the questions right and the least knowledgeable members get most (but not all) of the questions wrong.

Questions can be made more difficult by asking for finer discriminations or by asking about less well known subjects. 'Skimmed milk contains less fat than whole milk – True or False' is an easier question than 'Skimmed milk contains less fat than semi-skimmed milk – True or False' or 'Skimmed milk contains less calcium than whole milk – True or False'.

First of all decide what are the areas of knowledge that you wish to test. Box 9.2 is an example of how you might map out the points of information to be studied. Then write as many questions as you can (many more than you want to use in the final questionnaire) checking them against textbooks and other sources. Next discuss the questions with people who know a lot about the subject ('experts') and find out which questions they find confusing or irrelevant or where they disagree as to the right answer. Also discuss the questions with some people like those on whom you wish to use them and find out which questions they find difficult to understand or confusing. After these two sets of discussions, you will probably discard some questions, modify others and add some new ones.

The next stage is to give your questionnaire to a group who should be very knowledgeable and a group whose knowledge is expected to be poor. If the knowledgeable group does not score highly or the less knowledgeable group does not score low the questionnaire needs major revision.

The same data can be used to check each question for difficulty. If everyone gets it right it is too easy and if everyone gets it wrong it is too difficult. Questions should also be checked for discriminatory power. A good question is one which those who score highly on the whole questionnaire get right and those who score low get wrong. Another way of identifying useful questions is to look for questions which most of the experts get right and most of the less knowledgeable group get wrong. (In fact some of those who do not know the correct answer will be expected to get it right by guessing. The question of guessing and what score corresponds to no knowledge is discussed further at the end of this chapter.) The formal testing of questions is described in Box 9.5.

At the end of this process you will probably need to discard several more questions and modify others. Check that the questionnaire still covers all the areas of knowledge that you wish to measure.

Lastly it would be good to compare the scores from your questionnaire against the results from some other instrument that measures the same area of knowledge. Unfortunately very few validated instruments are available and so it may be impossible to find a suitable instrument for comparison.

This process has covered the validation steps described in Chapter 5. Face validity was checked by getting experts and users to scrutinise the questions; content validity by checking the questions covered all areas of knowledge initially mapped out; construct and criterion validity were checked by showing that experts scored higher than non-experts and by comparing the scores from your questionnaire with that of some other instrument. When you have done all these things you can be confident that you have produced a valid measure of this area of knowledge. All these validation procedures and a summary of their results should be included in the methods section of a full report of your study.

Box 9.5

Testing questions intended to measure nutrition knowledge

1 **Difficulty index**

Percent of respondents getting question correct. Generally select questions with a difficulty index between 25% and 75%.

2 **Discriminatory power**

a *Ratio of proportions correct in top and bottom quartile*

Score the whole questionnaire and identify people coming in top 25% overall (top quartile) and people coming in bottom 25% overall (bottom quartile).

For each question calculate:

TQ = proportion of people in top quartile who get question correct
BQ = proportion of people in bottom quartile who get question correct.

$$\text{Top bottom quartile index} = \frac{TQ - BQ}{TQ + BQ}$$

For the perfectly discriminating question this ratio will be 1 and in a totally non-discriminating question it will be 0.

Questions with a ratio of more than 0.3 are likely to be useful.

b *Cronbach's Alpha*

This is a more elaborate statistic to describe the consistency of the answers to an item (question) with the response to other items in the instrument.

Scoring knowledge questionnaires (some refinements)

So far we have been concerned with compiling a set of questions which measure knowledge. Usually we then want to combine the results to form a knowledge score. This is an example of constructing a multi-item instrument and raises several problems which were discussed in Chapter 6 (see Box 6.5). If the questions cover several different topics (e.g. fat, fibre, salt) then sub-scores for each of the different topics may provide more refined measures of knowledge. The simplest way to score questions is to give one mark for each correct answer. This however means that each question makes the same contribution to the knowledge score (has the same weighting).

There are three reasons why you may wish to make some questions contribute more than others to the final score. First you may have reason to regard some questions as more important and relevant to healthy eating than others. For example you may think that it is more important to know that 'Skim milk contains less fat than Whole milk' than 'Straight cut chips contain less fat than crinkle cut chips' (because the milk information is likely to have a greater impact on fat intake). Second you may feel that some questions are more difficult than others so that a higher score should be given for getting them right. Third you (or a statistician examining your results) may find some questions discriminate better than others and wish to attach more weight to them.

All these refinements can be allowed for by different scoring systems which give different marks to different questions (i.e. attach different weights). It may be helpful to discuss these possibilities with a statistician when you are developing your questionnaire to measure knowledge.

'Don't know' responses and failure to respond

Many respondents when they are not sure about the answer to a true-false question make no response. Some questionnaires use a 'don't know' response in addition to the 'true' and 'false' responses. This discourages guessing and allows people who feel they do not know the answer to make a positive response.

When a 'don't know' response is included wrong answers indicate incorrect knowledge and a score of 0% may be taken to indicate no knowledge. The problem with this approach is that 'don't know' responses or non-responses cannot be simply equated with no knowledge. People who know the right answer but do not have confidence in that knowledge may select the 'don't know' response. Also people who would choose the right answer if they thought about it may select the 'don't know' option as the response requiring least effort.

Guessing

One can attempt to get round the problem of 'don't know' and non-responses by not including a 'don't know' and asking respondents simply to guess the answer for any question if they do not know it. The instruction and layout of the questionnaire is designed to encourage the respondent to make a true or false response for every item. If someone who knows nothing guesses the answer randomly they will get a true-false answer correct about half the time. If they know the correct answer but are not very confident about it they are still likely to make a correct response.

If each correct answer scores one and each incorrect answer scores zero then those who know nothing will score about 50% so that 50% corresponds to a zero knowledge score. A score substantially below 50% indicates that they have incorrect beliefs. Scores around 50% may indicate either no knowledge (with all random guessing) or a combination of some correct knowledge and some incorrect beliefs.

The problem with this approach is that, while it may work well in an interview situation with a co-operative respondent, being asked to guess when you do not know the answer may seem against intuitive common sense. The respondent may therefore persist in making no response or even worse become irritated and decline to take part in your study at all.

The difficulties of interpreting and scoring 'don't know' responses have to be traded off against the difficulties which may be caused by trying to force all respondents into making a true or false response to every item. Neither solution is perfect.

Has knowledge been changed by a health promotion activity?

Often a promotion of healthier eating will have the objective of providing information. The items of knowledge to measure must be carefully selected to help you decide whether your activity has contributed to any change.

Suppose that the activity consisted of giving people a leaflet on how to reduce their risks of getting a heart attack. We could construct the questionnaire so that some questions covered items and examples mentioned in the leaflet while other questions covered items not mentioned in the leaflet. If the questions directly linked to items in the leaflet show more change than the other questions, this suggests that reading the leaflet had contributed to the change in knowledge.

In order to evaluate an activity intended to change knowledge of healthier eating you need to be able to answer the questions:
  'Has knowledge in the group changed?'
  'If it has changed, was this due to the promotion activity?'

The ways in which you might answer the second of these questions are discussed in the section on causal inference in Chapter 4.

What is the right answer – living with uncertainty

This chapter began by discussing the distinction between knowledge and belief. In order to classify a response as right or wrong we have to assume that there is a right answer to the question and that we know what it is. For topics like the nutrient content of foods or the chemical structure of nutrients there is little room for argument as to the right answer. When we come to the physiological function of nutrients and particularly to the dietary cause of disease there is much less agreement, while simple 'rules for healthy eating' are often disputed.

Examples of statements which would be universally agreed are:

    Unsaturated fatty acids contain double bonds.

    Ascorbic acid is Vitamin C.

    Skimmed milk contains less fat than whole milk.

    Wholemeal bread contains more fibre than white bread

    Sugar is added to some commercial brands of peanut butter.

Examples of statements about which some very well informed experts would be uncertain are:

    Eating less salt reduces your risk of getting high blood pressure.

    Eating more fruit and vegetables reduces your risk of getting colon cancer.

    Sugar in manufactured products contributes to obesity.

    People ought to eat something for breakfast.

    Brown rice is 'better' for you than white rice.

    Tartrazine is a cause of hyperactivity in children.

You will note that the examples about which there is no disagreement are generally rather trivial and less important for practical purposes. Some like those on chemical structure are not relevant to food choices affecting health. However, the examples about which there is some uncertainty are generally directly relevant to health and food choices.

Reducing the scope for disagreement

It is often possible to reduce the scope for dispute about the right answer by modifying the wording of statements. Consider these three statements:

    1   'We ought to eat less fat'

    2   'Most nutritional experts recommend that we should eat less fat'

    3   'The NACNE report recommended that we should eat less fat'.

The first statement could be described as a simple 'rule for healthier eating' and there is scope to argue whether it is correct. The third statement is undoubtedly correct and there is no room for dispute. However, the third statement tests detailed knowledge of an influential text while we are really concerned with eating behaviour. The second statement probably represents the best compromise.

This example suggests that in many cases it is better to settle for measuring beliefs relevant to eating and avoid the problem of trying to define nutritional knowledge. The first statement is the one which is most relevant to a person's food choices. The information which is needed to plan or evaluate a health promotion activity is how many people hold this belief and how strongly they hold it.

A further problem arises from the use of the word 'we'. The statement is based on general advice for the whole population but is not true for certain individuals

Box 9.6

Reference books for 'knowledge'

NACNE (1983). National Advisory Committee for Nutrition Education.
Proposals for Nutrition Guidelines for Health Education in Britain.
(London, Health Education Council). (Also known as the 'James Report'.)

COMA (1983). 'Diet and Cardiovascular Disease.'
Report on Health and Social Subjects 28. (London HMSO.)

US Department of Health and Human Services (1988).
Surgeon General's Report on Nutrition and Health (The Koop Report)
DHHS (PHS) Publications No. 88-50210. (Washington DC, US
Government Printing Office.)

National Research Council (1982).
Diet, Nutrition and Cancer. (Washington DC, National Academy Press.)

National Research Council (1989) 'Diet and Health.'
Implications for reducing chronic disease risk. (Washington DC, National
Academy Press.)

Gormley T. R., Downey G. & O'Beirne D. (1987).
Food, Health and the Consumer. (London Elsevier.)

Passmore R. & Eastwood M. A. (1986).
Human Nutrition and Dietetics. 18th Edition. (Edinburgh, Churchill
Livingstone.)

(for example those who are severely underweight or are already eating a very low fat diet). If someone responds that 'we should not eat less fat' it is unclear whether this is a correct assessment of their own nutritional need or an incorrect assessment of the general population (and their own) need.

The basis for valid knowledge

The difficulty in agreeing what is correct information and therefore true belief (knowledge) arises for two reasons. First we are always trying to compress complicated ideas and the results of years of study into simple and usable statements. Second in many areas of food knowledge there is still not enough information with which to settle the arguments. Furthermore even where information is agreed to be correct it is often not clear that it will be useful in trying to influence behaviour.

It is inconvenient to find that it is so difficult to agree what is knowledge in the field of healthy eating. However, we cannot stop promotion of healthier eating until all uncertainty is removed and unanimity is reached. The best practical approach is to take your 'knowledge' from well-known authoritative textbooks and reports on diet and health (see Box 9.6). Then check this 'knowledge' and its practical relevance with local people who are well informed on eating and health. This is as close as we can get to knowledge that will support eating choices that really are healthy. It is also the best foundation we can get for the construction of valid measures of relevant nutritional knowledge.

Would it be better to measure belief?

It is wise to remember that often when we think we are measuring knowledge we are actually measuring agreement with our own belief (opinion). Obsessive effort to avoid all areas where there is lack of unanimity among experts can divert us from exploring areas of information that are highly relevant to healthy eating. There is much to be said for asking respondents to agree or disagree with statements rather than to classify them as true or false. This avoids the problem of defining knowledge by treating it as belief. The measurement of belief is discussed in the next chapter.

Further reading

Link between knowledge and behaviour

Charny M. & Lewis P. A. (1987). 'Does health knowledge affect eating habits?'
    Health Education Journal 46, 172-176.

Instruments to measure knowledge

Mehrens W. A. & Lehmann I. J. (1978).
    Measurement and Evaluation in Education & Psychology (2nd edition). Publ.
    Holt, Rinehart & Winston.
    Chapter 9 Writing the objective test item: Short-Answer matching and true-false.
    Chapter 10 Writing the objective test item: Multiple choice and context
    dependent.
Prefontaine M. (1975). 'Construction and validation of a nutrition test.'
    Journal of Nutrition Education 7, 152-154.

Examples of nutritional knowledge measurement

Anderson A. S., Umpathy D., Palumbo L. & Pearson D. W. M. (1988). 'Nutrition knowledge assessed by a structured questionnaire in a group of medical patients.'
Journal of Human Nutrition and Dietetics 1, 39-46.

Clark M. B., Evans E. M. & Hamilton-Smith M. B. (1986). 'Doctors as nutrition educators.'
British Medical Journal 293, 928-931.
(This example includes a lot of the pitfalls discussed in this chapter.)

Tate J. U. & Cade J. (1990). 'Public knowledge of dietary fat and coronary heart disease.'
Health Education Journal 44, 32-35.

White C. W., Albanese M. A., Anderson E. E. & Caplan R. (1977). 'The status of cardiovascular health knowledge among sixth, seventh and eighth grade children.'
Circulation 56, 480-484.
(The relevance of the knowledge tested in this example to health behaviour is debatable.)

Examples of knowledge-based evaluation

Joffe M. (1988). 'Staff training for a food policy with built-in evaluation.'
Health Education Journal 46, 172-176.

Watson D., Moreton W. & Jessop E. G. (1988). 'Coronary awareness – Evaluation of a weeks' campaign.'
Health Education Journal 47, 47, 49-53.

Nichols, S., Waters W. E., Woolaway M. & Hamilton-Smith M. (1988). 'Evaluation of the effectiveness of a nutritional health education leaflet in changing public knowledge and attitudes.'
Journal of Human Nutrition & Dietetics 1, 233-238.

10 · Measurement of attitudes

Summary

Attitudes are one of many determinants of an individual's eating behaviour. An attitude has different components involving beliefs and values that interact with each other in a complex fashion. It is unrealistic to expect to measure these mental processes with single questions or to describe all the influences on eating with a few attitude scores.

Information on beliefs, credibility of information sources, values of health and other consequences of eating, food likings and intentions is needed in planning health promotion to judge whether possible strategies are likely (or unlikely) to be successful. This information is also useful for assessing the outcome of health promotion activity and giving insights as to how those outcomes were achieved.

Simple qualitative interviewing may be very helpful. Description of the frequencies of responses to opinion poll type questions can also be useful but the results have to be interpreted with care.

Introduction

The first part of this chapter briefly considers what attitudes are and their roles in why people choose particular eating behaviours. The next part considers which aspects of attitude are particularly important in planning or evaluating health promotion. The last part discusses methods which have been claimed to provide some information on attitudes.

What are attitudes?

The word 'attitude' is a vague and all-inclusive term for the ways of thinking that affect what a person does or says about different situations. An attitude is defined as a regularity in an individual's practical thoughts indicating something that is fairly consistent over time. A 'motive' is similar to an attitude but may not be so consistent over time. Psychologists have done a great deal of work on the complexities of the beliefs, values, intentions, impulses, likes and dislikes that comprise attitudes and motivation. Some important concepts are summarised in Table 10.1.

Table 10.1   Components of attitude and motivation

Cognitive factors – What you think
Beliefs and opinions   e.g. How strongly you are convinced that eating
                          fatty foods increases your risk of heart disease.

Affective factors – What you feel
Values and motives   e.g. How emotionally attached you are to
                          reducing your risk of heart disease.

Conative factors – What you deliberately want to do
Intentions   e.g. You now plan to eat less fried foods in the
                          future.

How you react without reasoning (consciously or not)
Impulses and cravings   e.g. You nibble at chocolates or potato crisps if
                          they are available.
Likes and dislikes   e.g. You particularly relish the taste and smell of
(Sensory preferences)   fried eggs.
                          You dislike the taste and mouth-feel of skimmed
                          milk.

Knowledge→Attitude→Behaviour: An unsatisfactory model of education

Traditional health education sought to change eating behaviour through increasing knowledge and spreading information about diet. The simplistic view was widespread that change in knowledge leads to change in attitude and then change in behaviour. Even today this is still the theory underlying some health promotion activity. There is however ample evidence that improvements in knowledge by themselves are not enough to influence behaviour or even to create interest in healthier eating.

The theory of reasoned action

The theory of reasoned action asserts that some eating behaviour of some people may be influenced to some extent by what they believe. If people believe that eating or not eating particular foods will improve their health they might alter their eating behaviour accordingly. However, a key extra condition must be present if a person's beliefs are going to affect their behaviour. They must not only believe that the behaviour will cause a health effect but also they must value that effect. For example someone may know which breakfast cereals are rich in fibre and know that eating more fibre will reduce their risk of getting bowel disease. Even so they will only choose fibre-rich breakfast cereals if they value reducing their risk of these diseases and value it sufficiently to accept the bother of finding and buying a different food and coping with a change in taste.

This theory is only part of the truth, even for the best educated and most rational people. Many food choices are made under other influences such as unreasoned attitude (I have never had it and I don't like it) or sheer habit. Also health considerations are only one among many possible reasons for acting (Table 10.2). Health reasons may conflict with other values such as eating what one's family and friends eat, eating cheaply, enjoying certain food flavours and so on.

It is certainly not true that increasing knowledge of healthy eating will by itself lead people to choose healthier eating. A realistic approach to health promotion should be based on a model including all components of rational behaviour and make allowance for non-rational motivation.

Table 10.2   Immediate influences on an individual's eating choices

Availability
    Convenience
    Expense

Sensory influences (Palatability)
    Appearance of food
    Taste and smell (flavour)
    Texture (feel in mouth)

Personal influences
    Feeling hungry: wish to be full
    Emotional eating; cravings
    Expecting to eat at mealtime

Social context
    Interpersonal factors
    Cultural norms

Rational considerations
    Improve fitness
    Help concentration, improve mood
    Give long term health and prevent disease

(Note: Health considerations may be least influential and so come at the bottom of the list)

Beliefs × Values→Intention

A reason for eating or not eating something comes from two components:

Cognitive – beliefs – factual expectation as to what will be the effect of eating
a particular food (outcome)
Affective – values – practical evaluation of how much that outcome is
wanted

These combinations of beliefs and values about food are expressed in intentions to eat in particular ways.

The properties of the model can be simply expressed in a formula like this:

Beliefs × Values→Intention

This model provides a basis for predicting the sorts of reasons for choosing certain foods in a population. The strength of people's beliefs and values can be measured. The interaction of these components is multiplicative, not additive. (Doubling the strength of either the belief or the values doubles the strength of the intention; if either component is zero, the intention is zero.)

The size of the belief component depends on how relevant it is to the intention and how strongly (with what conviction) it is held. The overall belief will include the circumstances or consequences of a particular eating behaviour and the ability of the individual to carry out the action.

The size of the value component will be zero if the person is neutral and could not care less about the result of the action. The value component may be positive or negative. It is positive if the person is for the believed consequences of the action and negative if they are against those consequences. The 'for' or the 'against' values can be weak or strong.

In trying to decide the likely effect of beliefs and values on eating intentions, it is important that all are equally relevant to the circumstances in which the eating is actually done. For example, suppose we are trying to predict whether an individual will deliberately choose a polyunsaturated margarine or butter. Their beliefs about the effects of eating polyunsaturated fats and butter fats on risks that they feel to their own health may be predictive to some degree. General beliefs about the consumption of fats and the health of populations that are unrelated to the individual's perception of their own risk are unlikely to be predictive at all.

Measurement of attitude

We have to work out (infer) people's attitudes from how they behave in a few different situations or more usually from how they answer a set of questions.

142

For example, we might infer someone's attitude to fried foods by observing their behaviour in a canteen (do they grimace when given a fried food?) and in a supermarket (do they avoid the bacon, sausage and lard counters?). Alternatively we could ask them questions such as: Do you like chips, bacon and fried eggs and/or crisps? do you think fried food is healthy? do you find frying a convenient way to cook? and so on. In this way we can study how they think and feel about fried food.

However, we can never be sure how well we are measuring a motive not to eat fried food in that person. Answers to questions about beliefs and values justifying behaviour may not always relate to real intentions, perhaps for some reason not mentioned by the respondent. Furthermore the best of intentions may not be realised. For example someone may intend to cut down on fry-ups but not manage it because they love fried food and have always eaten lots of it.

The practical limitations on what can be measured

The reason underlying attempts at attitude measurement in relation to healthier eating is the desire to understand the motivational processes that influence the individual in making food choices. The discussion earlier in this chapter has made it clear that these motivational processes are extremely complex networks of mental processes. It is quite unrealistic to assess the motivational structure of behaviours like choosing skimmed milk or cutting the fat off bacon by measuring a single entity called 'an attitude to cream in milk' or 'an attitude to fat on bacon'. The thousands of influences on all eating relevant to health cannot be measured with a small number of attitude scores.

Psychometricians have developed many multi-item instruments which measure 'attitudes' to various things. These instruments have generally been poor in predicting behaviour and are unlikely to be helpful in predicting eating behaviour. Some psychologists have developed general models of motivation networks (e.g. Belief $\times$ Value$\rightarrow$Intention) designed to be more predictive of deliberate food choices. These models require measurement of the attitude components with all the attendant complexities of scaling. In the future this approach may prove of some use in collecting information for planning or evaluating promotion of healthier eating. However, they will need extensive development work before they are ready for such applications.

What information about attitudes is helpful for health promotion?

The aspects of attitude which are practically useful in planning, monitoring and evaluating local health promotion activities are limited. It is usually sufficient to identify the general nature, direction and frequency of relevant attitudes without attempting detailed measurement. The aspects of particular interest are beliefs about food and health, credibility of sources of such information, values relating to food and health, other competing values and sensory likes and dislikes for food.

Later in this chapter various items are presented which have been claimed to be indicators of attitudes or elements in a mental networks. Items like these have been quite extensively used in surveys. It is important to remember that there is little evidence or theoretical reason to suggest that they really measure some influence on eating behaviour. They need to be interpreted with great care and treated with healthy scepticism.

Beliefs and opinions

It was explained in the previous chapter that there is no sharp dividing line between knowledge and belief. The truth of a convinced opinion is independent of the processes in the believer's mind. If we are trying to promote certain eating behaviour (that we regard as healthier) it is important to know what people believe to be the connection between that eating behaviour and health, disease and other outcomes. We need to know what beliefs are held regardless of their truth or falsity and we need to know how strongly they are held.

Health authorities were encouraged and helped to provide smoke-free areas in health premises by being shown that the vast majority of their staff (including the smokers) were in favour of greater restriction on smoking. Evidence of changing attitudes to driving after drinking alcohol and low alcohol alternatives encouraged brewers and pub licensees to provide a greater range of low alcohol and soft drinks. Similarly information relating to opinions about eating may encourage retailers and caterers to make more provision for healthy eating. Alternatively information of this type may warn you that people are not ready for a particular change in catering provision so that you would be wise to reconsider.

Perceived credibility of sources

People tend to trust certain sources of information believing messages from these sources, while distrusting and disbelieving others. If we know which sources are better believed (have high credibility) we can seek to use them to make our health promotion more effective. We can also avoid wasting resources on health promotion through widely distrusted channels. Box 10.1 gives an example of one study on this question.

It must be noted that there can be a great difference between what people say they trust and what they act on as though they trusted. The family doctor may be trusted but his advice on healthy eating is often not acted upon. Parents may be influenced in how they feed their children by the children's schoolmates but few parents would name them as a trusted source of information. A more sophisticated approach to assessing credibility of information sources is to survey what actions people have actually taken in response to similar information from different sources.

Values

Nearly all health promotion includes an element intended to influence values. This is most overt in the KAB (Knowledge Attitude Behaviour) model of health education and least obvious in community development and empowerment models. However, even when the stated objective of health education is no more than consciousness raising or value clarification, there is an implied objective of drawing attention to values favourable to health or strengthening the effect of these values. The open ended discussion or the trigger video are intended to make the participants consider health issues and implicitly to make them value health more highly when deciding what they might do.

Box 10.1

Perceived credibility of different sources of information

Here is a list of some of the places from which people get information about how to eat healthily.

Which of them would you believe?

Which of them have you ever acted on – that is changed your eating habits as a result of the information?

	% of Respondents	
	Would believe	Ever acted on
Doctors	90	31
Dieticians	72	8
Nutritionists	70	3
Government information	50	2
Society	46	4
Cookery books	43	2
Parents	38	6
School	29	2
Magazines	18	3
T.V.	17	2

From: British Nutrition Foundation (1984). Eating in the early 1980s.

Since the relations among health and other values have so much influence on eating behaviour, we need to know about them when planning health promotion activities and when monitoring their effectiveness. There may be strongly held values which mean that certain approaches which challenge them are unlikely to be successful. For example, bravado may be an important motive for some young men. Knowing that a habit (e.g. consuming large amounts of alcohol) is a risk to health may provide a reason for doing it rather than for not doing it. Alternative approaches (e.g. 'The strong say No') may have to be used. Information is useless unless it is received by people holding appropriate values.

Similarly, when evaluating health promotion activities, shifts in values may be an indication that our work is having some effect. Unfavourable value systems may explain why the results of a particular health promotion activity have been disappointing.

Values are measured by giving respondents more or less direct and concrete statements and asking them to react positively or negatively and more or less strongly to these statements. Examples of these statements are included in Box 10.2.

Likings and preferences

Food likings are another part of attitudes which are highly relevant to promotion of healthier eating. Information on likings will be helpful in planning health promotion activity. People are likely to be reluctant to eat less of foods that they like very much or to eat more of foods that they dislike very much. Liking for a food is a judgement that it is very good to eat. It depends on sensory features such as taste, smell and appearance but also involves other factors such as past experience of the food and the context in which it is eaten (Table 10.2).

Likings are particularly important when contemplating health promotion through changes in catering provision such as less frequent provision of chips with school meals, increased provision of salads in staff restaurants, or partial replacement of white bread with wholemeal in hospital. When a change of this type is contemplated, it is wise to assess the likings of the consumers to check if they are ready for the change.

Relatively unsophisticated direct questioning can give some indication of likings and preferences but yields rather unreliable data. A more realistic measure of likings and preferences is obtained by testing actual choices with real food samples in the context in which they would normally be eaten (consumer sensory and use tests). This sort of testing is usually too time consuming and expensive to be practical in a health promotion context. Nevertheless information on likely actual choices is crucial to successful promotion of healthier eating by means of menu choices. At least try it on your colleagues and family if you cannot apply consumer science to this issue.

Behavioural intent

It is often useful to ask people whether they intend to adopt a different eating pattern. Of course, not everyone who says they intend to do something actually does it, but their stated intentions are an indication that they might make a change. It may not predict action if it conflicts with other desires or circumstances.

Qualitative interviews

For many purposes, the best way of exploring attitudes is by open questions in semi-structured interviews. This can give you considerable insight into people's beliefs, values, likes and dislikes and allows you to probe areas of interest and follow up unclear or vague replies. You can describe the range and variety of common attitudes with this method. Interviews with twenty or so people with differing views from your district may be sufficient to give you a useful impression of what beliefs, opinions and values are held in the population and what shifts in these might be helpful. This type of data is therefore very useful.

It is however difficult to standardise the results of exploratory interviews and even more difficult to report the responses to a set of open-ended questions in a concise fashion. Doing qualitative interviews and reporting their results is a skilled task and interviewers have to be properly trained. Qualitative interviews are also time consuming so that you will usually have to restrict yourself to information from fairly small numbers of people. If it is important to collect information from larger numbers or representative samples then you will probably have to be content with the much less informative data obtainable from more structured techniques and closed questions. Even so, a few semi-structured interviews are invaluable in providing information needed to design and develop closed instruments (see Chapter 6).

Survey of attitudes – opinion polling

Attitudes can be assessed by using appropriately designed sets of questions. In designing questions the first point to be settled is whether you would be content with an indication of strength of opinion in the population or you really want to quantify the strengths of individuals' attitudes. The strength of opinion in the population can be estimated from the frequency of different responses to appropriate questions. This approach is sometimes described as 'Opinion Polling'. It must be contrasted with the more refined methods of attitude measurement necessary to explore individual motivation of food choices and other eating behaviour.

The following questions and response format illustrate opinion 'polling'.
Please indicate your agreement or disagreement with these statements:

It's just fate whether you get heart disease. You can't do anything about it.

Strongly
agree   Agree   Neither agree
                              nor disagree   Disagree   Strongly
                                                               disagree

You can reduce your risk of heart disease by watching how you eat.

Strongly
agree   Agree   Neither agree
                              nor disagree   Disagree   Strongly
                                                               disagree

Questions like this have been widely used. Other examples of 'opinion poll' type questions are shown in Box 10.2.

Box 10.2

Some opinion poll type questions which could be used in attitude surveys

1 Beliefs
* Please indicate for each of the things listed below how important you think it is in contributing to the development of heart disease:

	Very important	Important	Not very important	Not at all important	Don't know
Eating too much sugar	☐	☐	☐	☐	☐
Not eating regular meals	☐	☐	☐	☐	☐
Drinking too much alcohol	☐	☐	☐	☐	☐
Eating food containing a lot of animal fat	☐	☐	☐	☐	☐
Drinking coffee	☐	☐	☐	☐	☐
Eating too much salt	☐	☐	☐	☐	☐

Continued opposite

Box 10.2 (Continued)

* Please indicate below your answer to the following questions:

	Definitely no	Probably no	Probably yes	Definitely yes
Would eating wholemeal bread improve your health?	☐	☐	☐	☐
Would eating wholemeal bread improve your digestion?	☐	☐	☐	☐
Would eating wholemeal bread reduce your risk of heart attack?	☐	☐	☐	☐

Please say whether you agree of disagree with the following statements:

	Agree a lot	Agree a little	Disagree a little	Disagree a lot
To keep healthy you need to sit down to a proper meal at least once a day	☐	☐	☐	☐
It doesn't matter what you eat as long as you vary your diet a lot	☐	☐	☐	☐
Eating between meals is bad for your health	☐	☐	☐	☐
If you like something it means it's good for you	☐	☐	☐	☐

Continued overleaf

Box 10.2 (Continued)

2 Values

* Please indicate below your answer to each of the following questions:

	Not at all	A little	Moderately	Very much
How much do you value improving your health by eating wholemeal bread?	☐	☐	☐	☐
How much do you fear harming your health by eating fried food?	☐	☐	☐	☐
How much do you value reducing your risk of heart attack by eating wholemeal bread?	☐	☐	☐	☐
How much do you fear increasing your risk of heart attack by eating fried food?	☐	☐	☐	☐

3 Liking
Please circle one of the letters to indicate how much you like the following foods.

A   Like them so much that I eat them whenever I can

B   Like them enough that I eat them most of the times I can

C   Like them so little that I don't eat them even when I can

Chocolates	A	B	C
Boiled sweets	A	B	C
Crisps	A	B	C

Continued opposite

When compiling these types of questions there is little point in having more than four or five categories since the wording is crude. You need to consider whether you want an odd number of categories allowing a neutral response or an even number of categories forcing respondents to indicate some preference. A 'don't know' response may be informative but effectively introduces a different dimension into the responses. Response categories may be unimodal (e.g. very interesting...not at all interesting) or bimodal (e.g. very good for health...neither good nor bad for health...very bad for health).

When constructing lists of 'opinion poll' type questions the items need to be balanced so that a person with a particular attitude set would find a similar number of statements with which they agreed and statements with which they disagreed.

With this sort of question you are restricted to describing the frequencies of different response categories. On the other hand they are easy to understand. They are probably the best that can be obtained from representative samples for most purposes in planning and monitoring health promotion.

Suppose for example, you have set the objective that you wish to increase the numbers who believe that heart disease is to some degree preventable. You could ask the questions on preventability of heart attack of a sample of the population before and after the health promotion activity. You could then compare the responses and determine whether there had been a change in the response frequencies. This might indicate that there has been a shift of belief in the desired direction, but it could also arise from a shift in the meanings of people's responses.

The limitations of opinion polling

This format has many limitations. It is probably safe to assume that someone who disagrees has a different attitude from someone who agrees but it is far from clear that an individual who responds 'strongly agree' holds that belief more strongly than someone who responds 'agree'. The scale is an ordinal scale at most (see Box 6.2). It is not clear precisely what is being measured. Is it an attitude which influences behaviour? or merely a verbal reflection on a matter of topical interest? or something in between these two things?

Polls on voting intentions taken between elections have different meanings to polls on election eve. The meaning of polls on more complex issues such as opinions on food and health are also likely to be influenced by events. Thus 'opinion poll' type questions are a rather treacherous tool for comparing two different populations or the same population before and after an event. You may measure some change in response frequency but beware that such results have to be interpreted with great care.

From single questions to multi-item scales

So far we have discussed single attitude questions. Often we want to combine the answers to several questions (items) into a single summary measure (a multi-item scale). For example we might combine several questions on importance of healthy eating into a single global measure of favourableness to healthy eating. In this process a lot of detail will be lost (which may be important) but it may be it is easier to see underlying trends. Such multi-item scales are difficult to construct and validate. Furthermore their usefulness in predicting behaviour related to healthy eating is questionable. Generally they cannot be constructed from 'opinion poll' type questions. If you are contemplating using such a multi-item attitude scale you would be well advised to consult a psychometrician or psychologist (see section on multi-item scales in Chapter 6).

Further reading

Henderson M. E., Morris L. L. & Fitz-Gibbon C. T. (1987)
How to measure attitudes. Newbury Park, London, Sage Publications Ltd.

General discussion of attitudes

Ajzen I. (1988).
Attitudes, personality and behaviour. Milton Keynes, Open University Press.

Qualitative interviewing

Kreuger R. A. (1988).
Focus groups, a practical guide for applied research. Newbury Park, London, Sage Publications Ltd.

Applications of Belief × Value→Intention

Tuorila H. (1987).
Selection of milks with varying fat contents and related overall liking, attitudes, norms and intentions. Appetite 8, 1–14.

Shepherd R. & Stockley L. (1985).
Fat consumption and attitudes towards food with a high fat content. Human Nutrition: Applied Nutrition 39A, 431–442.

Attitudinal surveys

British Nutrition Foundation (1984).
Eating in the early 1980s. Attitudes and Behaviour: Main Findings. London, British Nutrition Foundation.

Heart Beat Wales (1985).
Technical Report No. 2. Welsh Heart Health Study: Protocol and Questionnaire. Health Promotion Authority for Wales.

11 · Methods for studying habitual food consumption and eating patterns (food frequency questionnaires and diet history)

Summary

Eating behaviour is complex but can be described in terms of eating patterns and amounts consumed. Eating patterns refer to habitual timing, sequences, and combinations of eating. In the past little attention has been paid to eating patterns though they are relevant to health.

There are two approaches to estimating habitual eating patterns and food consumption; (1) general habit methods which ask directly about usual practice without specifying any particular occasion and (2) specified time methods which record behaviour in a defined short period of time which is a sample of total long term behaviour. Specified time methods can be food accounting methods, retrospective methods or prospective methods. General habit methods can only be retrospective. This chapter discusses the use of the main general habit methods, food frequency questionnaires and diet histories to measure consumption and eating patterns.

A food frequency questionnaire can be used with large numbers and is quicker and easier than other methods. It can provide a very rough estimate of usual consumption especially when considered together with portion size. The diet history uses a combination of information gathering methods to build up a picture of habitual consumption.

Eating patterns can be extracted from sufficiently detailed records of foods consumed or they can be explored with suitable questions on general habit.

Introduction

Eating behaviour is complex. A full description would cover not only the total amount of food and drink consumed (food consumption) but also eating patterns. Eating patterns include the foods eaten, times and occasions on which they were eaten, sequences of food eaten, combinations of food, the intervals between eating and the amounts eaten on different occasions. Food consumption is the total amounts of foods consumed in a period of time and is the result of these behaviours.

155

Often nutritional theory has been concerned only with food consumption and has ignored eating patterns. There are many reasons for thinking this an inadequate way to describe the effects of eating and drinking on health. In many situations the eating patterns may have more influence on health than total consumption. The dietary causes of dental caries are an example (see Box 11.1). When trying to prevent dental caries, the intervals and sequences in which

---

Box 11.1

Dietary causes of dental caries

Production of acid
Dental caries is caused by acid attacking the teeth and demineralising them. The acid is produced by the action of bacteria in the mouth which ferment sugars and other carbohydrates. Sugars are the most important of the fermentable carbohydrates but other carbohydrates such as starch can also be fermented to produce acid. Eating patterns which increase exposure of the teeth to acid will increase the risk of caries.

The dietary factors which increase time exposed to acid are:

Sequence of foods
The food which tends to remain on the teeth is food eaten last on any eating occasion. Sugary foods eaten at the start of a meal or snack are therefore likely to cause less caries than such foods eaten as a snack or at the end of a meal.

Frequency of eating occasions
The amount of food left on the teeth is greatest immediately after eating and then decreases until the next eating occasion. If the intervals between eating occasions are short, the levels of fermentable carbohydrate and therefore of acid are likely to stay high.

Oral hygiene
Cleaning the teeth after a meal will reduce the level of fermentable carbohydrate (and bacteria). Foods eaten immediately before teeth cleaning are therefore unlikely to contribute to caries.

Total sugar consumption
While total sugar consumption is not directly related to dental caries, people who frequently consume sugar and therefore have high risk of caries will also have high total sugar consumption.

---

sugary foods are eaten are likely to be more important than the total amount eaten. Whether energy is taken between meals as well as at meals may be important for weight and there is some evidence that energy consumed between meals can contribute to difficulties in weight control. Fourteen units of alcohol consumed over a week sounds reasonable but if it is all consumed in an hour or two it might represent a health problem.

Measuring the health relevant eating patterns as well as the total amounts consumed is therefore an important part of monitoring food policies.

Methods of estimating food consumption and eating patterns

Food consumption and eating pattern survey methods can be divided into three groups: food accounting methods, retrospective methods and prospective methods (Table 11.1). Food accounting methods estimate only consumption and cannot give information on eating patterns. They estimate consumption by recording what food is removed from store or sold and are mostly used to estimate consumption of groups rather than of individuals. Retrospective methods require the subjects to remember what they ate either in the immediate past or over a longer period. Prospective methods involve recording food at the time it is eaten. Retrospective methods are often referred to as 'Recall' methods and prospective methods as 'As eaten' methods.

Table 11.1 Methods of estimating food consumption and eating patterns

1 Food accounting methods
  (a) Food production and marketing information
  (b) Larder inventories

2 Retrospective methods (also called Recall methods)
  (a) 24-hour recalls
  (b) Diet history method
  (c) Food frequency questionnaires

3 Prospective methods (also called As Eaten methods)
  (a) Weighed inventory
  (b) Diet diaries – using household measures
  (c) Observation methods

Note: The diet history method (see page xx) and the National Food Survey (see Box 12.8) involve a mixture of these method types.

The retrospective and prospective methods have mostly been developed and used to study consumption but they could be used to study eating patterns. The next section will consider measurement of consumption. Measurement of eating patterns will be described in the last section of this chapter.

The concept of habitual consumption

Dietary influences on health generally act over decades or years rather than days or weeks. We are therefore interested in average consumption over a long period of time. This is referred to as habitual consumption. There is some vagueness about this concept since it is unclear whether it refers to mean consumption, modal consumption, median consumption or some other undefined summary measure. (The terms modal, median and mean are defined in Box 16.3.)

The time focus

All the methods listed in Table 11.1 estimate habitual food consumption but they can be divided into two sets. One set of methods directly estimates habitual consumption by considering consumption habits in general without reference to particular occasions (general habit methods). The other does so indirectly by considering actual consumption in a defined short time period (specified time methods).

The distinction between these two approaches is best understood by asking the question 'For which particular days did you estimate food consumption?'. For general habit methods the question cannot be answered because the estimate was not made for any particular day or occasion. For the specified time methods you can state exactly for which dates you estimated food consumption.

Generalisations over time are being made in both methods. In the general habit methods, the subject is left to create the generalisation from their experience using unspecified rules. In the specified time methods the investigator creates the generalisation by assuming that the time period studied was representative. General habit methods are likely to underestimate infrequent eating behaviour and so may estimate modal (commonest) consumption whereas specified time methods usually estimate mean consumption.

The distinction between general habit and specified time methods is not absolute but the food frequency questionnaire, diet history and related methods are predominantly used as general habit methods. These will be discussed in this chapter. The 24-hour recall, the diet diary and the weighed inventory are specified time methods and will be discussed in the next chapter. The food accounting methods applied to individuals will also be briefly discussed in the next chapter.

Should you choose a general habit or specified time method?

The general habit methods are based on the assumption that respondents can make a useful generalisation about their food consumption over many occasions and a long period of time. The theoretical basis for the method is as sound as that assumption. In practice, once designed, general habit methods are relatively easy for the subject to use, but their initial design is difficult.

The specified time methods are attractively simple in theory because it is clear what the 'true' results (namely what was consumed in that time period) should be. The fundamental weakness of the method comes in the next step which requires the crude assumption that the consumption in this specified time period is equal to the habitual consumption.

The specified time methods are difficult in practice. A great deal of effort has been put into developing methods of estimating the type and amount of food actually consumed in the specified period either retrospectively or prospectively. These methods demand a lot of co-operation from subjects and are time consuming and expensive to use. Prospective methods increase the accuracy of the information on actual consumption in the specified time period by collecting it at the time the food is eaten. Unfortunately this process is likely to disturb eating habits so that the food consumption which is so laboriously recorded is not representative of habitual consumption.

There is no satisfactory 'gold standard' method for habitual consumption; so methods cannot easily be criterion validated. The exceptions to this statement are those nutrients where consumption and output are normally in balance. In these cases measures of output (urinary excretion for sodium or double isotope method for energy) can be used as a criterion.

Reasons for collecting data

Data may be collected to answer four basic types of questions about food consumption (intakes, frequencies, amount on one occasion, sequences, etc.).
1   Is there a difference in food consumption between groups?
2   What is the mean consumption and distribution of consumption in a group?
3   Where is an individual in the rank order of food consumption in a group?
4   What is the absolute value of food consumption for an individual?

The first two questions are concerned with group values not individuals. Issues of this type are often important for health promotion. For example 'What is the mean percent of energy derived from fat in the group and what proportion of them derive 30% or less of their energy from fat?' and 'Is this group eating more wholemeal bread after compared to before the health promotion?'. The third type of information may be required when asking questions such as 'Do the people who have the best knowledge of health effects of fat have the lowest intakes of fat? (Are knowledge about fat and fat intake inversely correlated?)' The fourth type of question is usually only important in clinical studies.

For the first question neither random nor systematic errors matter (so long as there is no bias between the groups being compared). For the second question random error is not crucial but we must avoid systematic error as far as we can. For the third question systematic error is unimportant but random error must be minimised. For the fourth question both random and systematic error must be avoided as far as possible. (Types of error are defined in Box 5.5.)

Food frequency questionnaires

Food frequency questionnaires can be used to obtain information on what foods are being eaten, how often and (if portion sizes are estimated) how much. They are probably the only feasible method for studying food consumption by very large numbers of people.

The choice of foods to be included in a food frequency questionnaire depends on the purpose of the study. If you are particularly interested in consumption of certain foods or certain classes of food then the questionnaire will obviously include these. Chapter 13 discusses what foods to include if you are really trying to study nutrient consumption rather than food consumption.

Food frequency questionnaires are mostly used to enquire about eating without reference to any particular occasion and are therefore a general habit method. The questions should be introduced by a realistic time restriction such as 'Think about how you usually ate over the last three months'. If this time period is made very short (for example 'Think about what you ate last week') they can be used to enquire about eating in a defined short time period and the method merges into a specified time method.

To lump foods or to split them?

When presenting results it is convenient to lump similar foods into groups such as meat and meat products, dairy products and vegetables but should we ask questions in these terms? 'How often do you eat meat or meat products?' may make sense to the dietician but does the person eating black pudding, steak and kidney pie, chicken nuggets or sausage rolls think of them as 'meat products'? It is not easy to add together all the separate occasions on which you ate a set of what seem to be very different products. Initial interviews are helpful in showing what groupings are natural for respondents.

Some groupings would be nutritionally inappropriate. For example the fibre content of a portion of peas is much higher than that of a portion of lettuce. It is not right to lump them together under the heading 'vegetables' if you are interested in fibre intake.

Such considerations may lead you to split the questions and ask about foods individually rather than in groups. Instead of asking 'How often do you eat vegetables (other than potatoes)?', you might go to the opposite extreme and ask 'How often do you eat carrots?, How often do you eat parsnips?', and similar questions for turnips, swedes, other root vegetables, sprouts, cauliflower, cabbage, other green leafy vegetables, beans, peas, lettuce, tomatoes, onions and so on. This would make a very long questionnaire however. People would be likely to get bored by it and therefore complete it less accurately.

Also, if you add together the frequencies with which the different vegetables are eaten, the total for all vegetables will be much greater than the answer you get when you ask the question 'How often do you eat vegetables?'. When foods are lumped, the rare foods are liable to be forgotten leading to an underestimate. When they are split there is a tendency to overestimate low frequencies, leading to an overestimate of total consumption.

A compromise has to be made between the desire for greater detail and the desire to push answers into convenient looking groups. At an early stage you will decide roughly how long you want your questionnaire to be and this will limit how much you can split your food groups. Avoid groupings which combine foods that are usually eaten in different circumstances. For example 'sugar and preserves' is confusing because, although the two are very similar in nutritional terms, people do not use jam and sugar for similar purposes when eating. Similarly, salad vegetables and cooked leafy vegetables should probably not be combined since they are eaten in different situations.

Asking about frequency

Open questions might be used to ask about frequency as 'How many times a week do you eat chips?' but it is more usual to ask closed questions, such as:

How often do you eat chips?	A	Every day
	B	5-6 times a week
	D	2-4 times a week
	D	Once a week
	E	Less than once a week

Using a closed question like this indicates to the respondent the level of detail one is expecting in the answer and makes the information much easier to process. On the other hand it limits the information obtained. This question, for example, could not distinguish someone who never ate chips and someone who regularly ate them once a fortnight.

161

In designing closed questions it is important to produce appropriate response categories. For some studies we want response categories which will divide the population into groups and do not combine people with important differences into the same category. If we were asking about a food which is eaten frequently (such as bread in a traditional British diet), the response categories used in the chips question would be inappropriate because very few people would come into categories D and E. Similarly, if we were asking about food which is usually eaten infrequently such as kippers, these response categories would be inappropriate because nearly everyone would come into category E.

Increasing the number of response categories or using different response categories for different foods enables you to obtain more detail. On the other hand it also makes the questionnaire more difficult to complete, increasing the errors and even failures to respond.

Estimating portion size and quantity consumed

Certain foods are consumed in fairly standard portion sizes so that one can ask about number of portions consumed rather than frequency of consumption. Examples of such questions are:

How many slices of bread do you eat in a typical day?
How many oranges do you eat in a typical week?
How many eggs do you eat in a typical week?

For other foods it may be possible to estimate portion size with questions such as:
How many teaspoons of sugar do you put in your tea?
When you have potatoes how many do you usually eat?
Do you spread butter or marge on your bread,
A) thickly   B) medium   C) thinly?

One can attempt to improve the quantity estimate from these questions by asking additional questions about the size of the unit such as 'Do you have a level or a heaped teaspoon of sugar?' and 'What size are the potatoes that you eat?'. If the questions are being administered by interview, then you can use the methods for improving quantity estimates described in Box 12.3.

In other situations it may be possible to obtain an estimate of quantities by asking about weekly purchase. The answers to this type of question are however, difficult to interpret when several members of a household share the same purchases. Examples of these sorts of questions are:
How many pints of milk do you order each day?
How many pounds of butter do you buy each week?

It can be seen that the sorts of question illustrated in this section yield only the crudest estimates of quantity consumed.

162

Qualitative questions

For some foods it is as important to know what type is being eaten as it is to know how much is being eaten. Table 11.2 lists some foods where the type eaten may be of particular interest as markers of people's interest in healthier eating.

Table 11.2 Foods where type eaten is relevant to health concern

Bread	White, soft grain, brown, Hovis, wholemeal, etc.
Milk	Full fat, semi-skimmed, skimmed etc.
Yellow spreads	Butter, hard marge, soft marge, polyunsaturate rich marge, low fat spread etc.
Breakfast cereal	Cornflakes, Rice Crispies, Sugar Puffs, muesli, porridge, Shredded Wheat, Puffed Wheat, Weetabix, All Bran, Bran Flakes, Oat Crunchies, etc.
Preserves	Ordinary jam or sugar-reduced fruit spreads (jam).
Yoghurt	Natural, flavoured (sweetened), low fat, etc.
Tinned fruit	Canned in syrup, canned in fruit juice.
Rice	White or brown
Fizzy drinks	Ordinary or low calorie.

Questions on cooking methods may also give useful information for estimating intakes of fat, salt, vitamin C, etc. An example of such a question is:

'When you cook sausages,   A   Fry them with added fat
    do you usually?   B   Fry them without added fat
    C   Grill them with added fat
    D   Grill them without added fat'

Checklists of foods eaten yesterday

A simplified variant on the food frequency questionnaire and 24-hour recall methods (see Chapter 12) gives a list of foods and asks 'Which of these foods did you eat yesterday?'. It has the advantage over conventional frequency instruments of being very much easier to complete (young children can manage it). It may be less susceptible to memory and averaging errors than questionnaires which ask about 'usual' eating patterns. The very short time focus and the assumption that a food was eaten only once means it is not a reliable guide to an individual's eating pattern (unless administered on several different days to each individual) but it could be used as a guide to eating patterns of groups of people.

163

Dietary change questions

Another approach to monitoring food consumption is to ask whether eating habits have changed rather than attempt to measure the actual food consumption. Examples of the questions used in this approach are:

Since last year have you changed the amount of fish you eat?
- A) Eating more now
- B) Eating same amount
- C) Eating less now

Since last year have you changed the amount of fresh fruit you eat?
- A) Eating more now
- B) Eating same amount
- C) Eating less now

This type of question may offer an easy way of monitoring a food policy but it should be noted that these questions may be measuring attitudes (the perceived desirability) to dietary change as much as actual behavioural change.

Social acceptability bias

There is a risk that people may report consumption frequencies that they think are healthy or socially acceptable (for example under-reporting of alcohol consumption and over-reporting of fresh fruit consumption) rather than their actual consumption frequency. This applies to all methods including the food frequency questionnaires. Arranging for the questionnaire to be completed anonymously may reduce the problem but does not totally overcome it.

Food frequency questionnaires have to be designed so as to minimise this source of error. For example it was shown that changing the title on the questionnaire from 'food survey' to 'health survey' increased the reported frequency of consumption of foods viewed as 'healthy'.

The specified time methods, both retrospective and prospective, do not entirely avoid this bias. The bias when specific occasions are reported may be less than when a generalisation about habit is made. For example people may well answer the question 'How many pints of beer did you drink last night?' more accurately than the question 'How many pints of beer do you usually drink in a night?'.

Fully structured interviews

The previous sections have used the term 'questionnaire'. However, the same questions could equally well be asked in a fully structured interview. This would make it easier to ensure that the respondent answered all questions and would provide an opportunity to check the attentiveness of the respondent and the correctness of any unexpected answers.

Dietary history

Diet histories are a semi-structured interview that aims to discover the habitual food intake of individuals. Several different ways of taking a diet history have been described. Many investigators claim to use the Burke method of dietary history but most do not follow all the procedures she described. Usually the interview starts with a combination of a 24-hour recall and questions on habitual practice to establish an overall eating pattern. The second part of the interview uses a 'cross-check' list of foods which is used to ensure no items have been omitted. Information on likes and dislikes, food purchasing and uses of food is also collected to verify and clarify information obtained in the first part of the questionnaire. The method has the advantage that a professional effort is made to interpret, collate and compare the results of three or four styles of eliciting information from an individual. It is reasonable to hope that in the right hands the extra time taken yields better quality information than any single style on its own.

Discussion of where to conduct interviews and other practical aspects will be found at the end of the next chapter.

Measuring eating patterns

The discussion so far has concentrated on food frequency and quantity but this last section concentrates on measurement of eating patterns. As with consumption, eating patterns can be studied using either 'general habit' or 'time specified' methods.

All of the information needed to estimate habitual timing, sequence, combination or amount per occasion can in principle be obtained from 24-hour recall, weighed inventory or diet diary data. However, in practice records obtained by these methods have very rarely been used in this way. Often the necessary data are omitted or written only in rough form. For example, the times of a meal or drink should be recorded to the nearest 10 minutes at least.

Ideally the time of start and finish of each course or item should be recorded to the nearest minute. The group of foods in a course and the sequence of courses, foods and drinks should also be preserved in the record. Then so long as portion sizes can also be estimated for the period recalled, everything in the way of amount, frequency and pattern can be estimated for the period recalled or recorded.

Eating patterns can be explored with 'general habit' questions which do not refer to specific occasions. Examples of such questions are:
On a typical weekday how many main meals do you have?
How often do you eat sweets between meals?
Do you add sugar to tea? How many teaspoons?

Do you usually eat breakfast in the morning?
Do you usually have a cooked meal at lunchtime?
Do you usually eat as a family at lunchtime?
What time do you usually have your evening meal?
Do you usually have a drink at bedtime?
Do you usually have something to eat mid-morning?

Questions about specific eating occasions can also be used to explore eating or drinking patterns. For example:
Think about the last time you had an alcoholic drink:
Where was that? – Were you alone or with other people? – What were the circumstances? – What did you drink? – How much?

General habit and time specified questions may be used in combination. Box 11.2 is an example of questions used to investigate the frequency and energy content of drink breaks.

Box 11.2

Questionnaire for estimating frequency and energy content of drink breaks

We can talk about snacks in the sense of quick, light but rounded meals (these would have at least 2 or 3 items of food and drink). We can call these SUBSTANTIAL SNACKS.

Another way we can talk about snacks refers to when we have a drink, especially rich drinks like milk or alcohol, maybe with a biscuit, crisps or other snackfood. When this sort of snack happens we can call it a DRINK BREAK.

On a typical weekday how many MEALS and SUBSTANTIAL SNACKS do you have? (ring one number)

0   1   2   3   4   5   6   7   8   9   10   More than 10

On a typical weekday how many times do you have drinks OTHER than at meals or substantial snacks, i.e. how many DRINK BREAKS do you have a day? (ring one number).

0   1   2   3   4   5   6   7   8   9   10
11   12   13   14   15   More than 15

Continued opposite

Box 11.2 (Continued)

Thinking about what you have at DRINK BREAKS please describe as fully as possible what you had to drink and to eat (if anything) on the last occasion of this type.

LAST occasion of taking any sort of drink between Substantial Snacks or Meals.

Time of day

What you had to drink
Type of drink(s) (e.g. Coffee, Lemonade)
Brand name(s) of drink (e.g. Nescafe, Guinness)
How much of each type of drink (e.g. pints, cans, cupfuls)
Was milk added to the drink? Yes or No.
      If YES, how much milk?
      What type of milk (e.g. whole, semi-skimmed, skimmed)?
Was sugar added to the drink? Yes or No.
      If YES, how much sugar?

What you had to eat with your drink(s) (if anything)
Type of food(s) (e.g. crisps, biscuits)
Brand name(s) (e.g. Kit-Kat)
How much.

Now please describe as fully as you can the NEXT TO LAST occasion of this type.

NEXT TO LAST occasion of taking any sort of drink between Substantial Snacks or Meals.

Time of day.

What you had to drink [etc. etc., as above for last occasion].

The validation and use of this quiz are described in Blair *et al.* 1989.

Note combination of questions. Questions on frequency of meals and drink breaks are general habit questions. Questions on content of drink breaks are specified occasion questions.

Further reading

General Methods

Cameron M. E. & Van Staveren W. A. (1988).
Manual of Methodology for Food Consumption Studies. (Oxford University Press).
Chapter 4 'Purposes of food consumption studies.'
Chapter 6 'Methods for data collection at an individual level.'

Food frequency questionnaires

Willet W. C., Sampson L., Stampfer M. J. *et al.* (1985). 'Reproducibility and validity of a semi-quantitative food frequency questionnaire.'
American Journal of Epidemiology. 122, 51-65.

Shepherd R., Farleigh C. A. & Land D. G. (1985). 'Estimation of self-intake questionnaire.'
Appetite 6, 219-233.

Jain M., Howe G. R., Johnson K. C. & Miller A. B. (1980). 'Evaluation of a diet history questionnaire for epidemiological studies.'
American Journal of Epidemiology 111, 212-219.

Dietary history

Burke B. S. (1947). 'The dietary history as a tool in research.'
Journal of the American Dietetic Association 23, 1041-1046.

Food patterns

Southgate D. (1990). 'Nibblers, gorgers, snackers and grazers.'
British Medical Journal 300, 136-137.

Blair A. J., Booth D. A., Lewis V. S. & Wainwright C. J. (1989). 'Relative success of official and informal weight reduction techniques.'
Psychology and Health 3, 195-206.

12 · Methods for studying food consumption (specified time methods)

By A. Bone

Summary

Twenty-four hour recall is used to estimate food consumption retrospectively. This does not involve any disturbance in usual eating pattern but is subject to all the problems associated with relying on memory of past events.

Prospective methods avoid the problems of memory but suffer from the drawback that the process of recording what is eaten may well disturb the usual pattern of eating. The weighed inventory gives accurate information on quantity of food eaten in the defined time but is demanding on subjects and very disturbing of usual consumption. The food diary method with household measures gives less accurate information on quantity but demands less of subject and disturbs the usual consumption less.

Food accounting methods estimate consumption from food removed from store. This is usually applied to households rather than individuals.

The practical aspects of using these methods such as time and staff required are explored.

Introduction

This chapter describes the different methods that are available for studying food consumption in a defined time period. These methods are 24-hour recall, weighed inventory, diet diaries, observation and food accounting. It briefly describes what is involved and the advantages and disadvantages of each method.

Retrospective measurement (recall)

Retrospective methods collect information on food consumption by recall; that is, people are asked to remember what they have eaten at some time previously. A major advantage of these methods is that they require a lesser degree of subject co-operation than prospective methods, so that response rates may be better. They also have the advantage that unlike the prospective methods they do not interfere with spontaneous food choices and eating. Higher response rates and non-interference with eating will both tend to increase the validity of these methods. A further advantage of these methods is that they require less staff time. However, a major disadvantage is that the data collected are entirely based on the respondent's memory.

24-hour recall

Subjects are asked to recall all food and drink consumed over the preceding 24 hours. The accuracy of this method relies on the ability of the respondent to remember what they have eaten and on them being able to describe quantities of food taken. Accuracy can be improved by using food models and household measures as discussed in the section on food diaries (Box 12.3). The validity of the method can also be improved by interviewing techniques that prompt memory of eating and drinking occasions without introducing bias. Detailed information on the collection of a 24-hour recall can be found in Box 12.1.

Nutrient intakes can vary greatly from day to day however. It is therefore generally accepted that a single 24-hour recall is a poor guide to the usual intake of an individual. Repeated 24-hour recalls on the same individual will give a much better indication of their usual intake. There is more discussion on how many days are needed to estimate habitual intake in Box 12.4. Single 24-hour recalls can nevertheless be used to estimate the mean intake of a population group and to establish differences between groups.

Recalls over a period of time longer than 24 hours are sometimes used but should be viewed with even greater suspicion since they rely on the subject's memory over a long period including more than one example of each meal time. Can you remember what you had for supper seven days ago?

Prospective measurement ('as eaten')

Methods of measuring food intake prospectively (i.e. as eaten) have the major advantage of reducing reliance on memory and recall errors. Because subjects are meant to record food at the time they eat it there is less chance of them forgetting or misreporting what they have eaten. With prospective methods it is also possible to improve the estimation of quantity by including weighing in the procedures.

However, they have a number of drawbacks. Firstly, the process of recording makes the subject very aware of what they are eating and this is liable to interfere with their 'usual' food intake. Secondly, methods involving recording and especially weighing require a high level of subject co-operation and hence will have a lower response rate. Thirdly they require more investigator time. Lastly all the prospective methods have to sample a relatively short time period and this may not reflect habitual eating over some months.

Box 12.1

How to conduct a 24-hour recall

The aim of a 24-hour recall is to get accurate information on the food eaten during the previous day.

Time period covered
The information is collected on the 24 hours including and preceding the last main meal.

What is recorded
Everything eaten or drunk should be recorded, even if it is a small amount.

Subjects often only volunteer information on meals consumed, and probing questioning will be needed to ensure all snacks, sweets, nibbles and sips are recalled.

How to ask the questions
Always use open questions. Begin by asking 'What was the last (most recent) thing that you ate or drank?' rather than a leading question such as 'Did you eat breakfast today?'. Follow on with 'What did you have before that?'. Do not ask 'What did you have for lunch (tea, dinner, supper, mid-morning)?'.

Recall of eating will be much improved if it is linked to non-eating activities by use of prompts such as:
   'What were you doing at this time?'
   'Where did you go?'
   'Who was with you?'
   'Did you have something to eat at the station/on the train/in the coffee room, etc?'.

Check questions
Check the time foods were eaten. This makes it easier to identify gaps of time.

Check details about the food consumed again by using open questions, for example:
   'Did you have anything on it?'
   'How was it cooked?'
   'What kind of . . . . was it?'

Check for leftovers and seconds

Ways of improving estimates of portion size are shown in Box 12.3.

Prospective methods trade off the invalidating effect of interfering with usual eating habits against greatly decreased recall errors and the accuracy which comes from weighing. The balance of advantage in this trade off is difficult to establish.

The weighed inventory method

When collecting a weighed inventory the subject weighs and writes down each item of food or drink as they consume it. The food is weighed in the form in which it is to be eaten (i.e. after it has been cleaned and cooked). Any left-overs are weighed and written down at the end of a meal. Individual components of combined dishes need to be weighed. For example if the subject eats a sandwich they will need to record the weight of the bread, the weight of the butter or margarine, and the weight of the filling. For complicated items such as a casserole, the subject is usually asked to weigh the item whole, but also to record detailed information about the quantities of ingredients used, method and time of cooking, and number of portions served so that its contents can be calculated later. Figure 12.1 shows an example of a completed record.

DAY/DATE: MONDAY MAY 5th.

RECORDING DAY CODE: MOND.
RECORDING DAY NO: RS

TIME	FOOD/DRINK	WEIGHT SERVED	LEFT OVERS	BRAND/RECIPE ETC.	TIME	CODE	AMOUNT
9:30	GRAPEFRUIT	119		— Tinned - syrup.	0930	0742	0119
	APPLE JUICE	134			0930	0775	0134
2-00	CHOC BISCUIT	16		- Organic	1200	0058	0016
2-00	SCRAMBLED EGG.	66		2 egg, marg ~ 2tb milk,	1400	0173	0066
	BREAD	38		- White	1400	0033	0038
	MARGARINE	16		OUTLINE	1400	0186	0016
	SALMON	27		Tinned	1400	0498	0027
	CRISPS	6			1400	0652	0006
	WHITE WINE.	121			1400	0907	0121
5:45	CHICKEN.	58		Roast - meat only No skin ~ bone.	1745	0221	0058
	BAKED POTATO	183			1745	0643	0183
	PEAS	64		frozen - boiled	1745	0623	0064
	ONION SAUCE.	53		Bisto · Granules	1745	0927	0053
	WHITE WINE.	116			1745	0907	0116
10:00	WHITE WINE	121			22-00	0907	0121
NOTES:							

Figure 12.1 **Example of page from a weighed inventory record book**

In theory all food items should be weighed. However, in practice certain food items such as sweets, packets of crisps, commercially produced biscuits and cakes, and drinks in public houses are eaten in standard weight portions and need not be weighed before recording. In situations where weighing cannot be carried out conveniently, for example restaurant meals, a detailed description of the foods eaten including descriptions of portion sizes is usually obtained so that weights of items can later be estimated by the investigator.

Frequent contact with the fieldworker and careful checking of records allows probable missing information to be detected. Incomplete description of foods can often be spotted or unaccounted time gaps when foods may have been eaten. The fieldworker can then use recall methods to obtain this information and correct the record. This is particularly useful when the subject forgets to write down items of food which is the commonest source of under-recording errors. Other strategies to ensure all foods consumed have been weighed and recorded include asking the subject to collect wrappers of 'snack' items like crisps and packets of sweets and chocolate. This approach is particularly useful when collecting records from children.

Inevitably there will be occasions when food items or complete meals have not been weighed. The number of estimated weights acceptable in a record should be decided prior to commencing a survey. A typical rule could be to discard records of days where the weight of more than 20% of the food items is estimated and to discard the complete records where more than three out of seven days' records have to be discarded.

Methods involving weighed records have the disadvantage that weighing everything you eat and writing it down is very tedious for the subject. This means that a high degree of co-operation is required from the respondent and there is a danger of low response rates with their attendant bias. Although many subjects are surprisingly co-operative the method is clearly unsuitable for those who have difficulty with writing or weighing or are confused. Frequent contact and a good relationship with the fieldworker throughout the inventory period will help to maintain the subject's motivation. For this reason it is important that the fieldworker is not in a rush but has time to talk with the subjects; 'friendly' time for this purpose must be allowed in the fieldwork schedules.

The major disadvantage of the weighed inventory method is that the acts of weighing and recording may themselves alter eating patterns (consciously or subconsciously) and amounts of food consumed. The fieldworker can only attempt to minimise this error by impressing on the subject that they should try to choose foods and eat them in their usual manner.

If you are planning a study using the weighed inventory method it is a good idea to discuss your plans with your local dietician and with an established survey team at an early stage. Further advice on the equipment and personnel needed is given in Box 12.2. The people needed to run a survey are discussed later in this chapter.

Box 12.2

Practical considerations for using the weighed inventory method

Weighing scales
Accurate scales are essential. Ordinary household scales are not good enough. Electronic scales with digital read-out, accurate to ±2g are ideal. Depending on the quality of the scales prices vary from £25-£100 each. It is often possible to borrow scales from larger survey teams.

Most electronic scales have a taring system so that the scales can be zeroed after each item of food has been added to the weighing plate. This can cause confusion and with some groups of subjects it is better to teach 'cumulative' weighing rather than taring.

Before starting a study it is essential to check the calibration of each set of scales using standard weights.

Record books
The design of record books should be kept simple.
The record book should include simple written instructions on the weighing procedure, on the recording of information, and about coping with 'unweighed' food items.
An example of a day's record should be given.
The design of recording form is important. It should include columns for:

1 Recording the time a food item is eaten
2 A description of the food
3 Description of recipes or brand names
4 The weight served
5 The weight of left overs
6 Columns to be completed by study workers showing food codes, corrected weights, etc.

It is usually better to provide record forms as a booklet rather than individual sheets which can be easily lost. Booklets should be about an A5 size as this is easy to carry around.

Combined weighing and recording systems
There are sophisticated systems (such as the PETRA system) that combine electronic scales and automatic recording facilities. This means that the user does not have to make a written record but just has to describe each food item as they weigh it. This can be useful with subjects who find writing difficult and it may reduce the problem of under-recording. These systems are expensive to buy.

Continued opposite

The diet diary (household measure or unweighed food record)

A less demanding method of collecting food records is to ask the subject to write
down everything they eat or drink but instead of weighing each item to describe
the quantities eaten in household measures (e.g. a bowlful of soup, a glass of
milk, two tablespoonfuls of rice). This method is much less accurate than
weighing but has the compensating advantages of less disturbance of the usual
eating pattern and probable higher response rates from the study sample since it
is less demanding of the subjects.

Although somewhat easier for the subject this technique is more demanding for
the fieldworker who has to use a great deal of skill in estimating weights from the
descriptions of food consumed. Sometimes the fieldworker will ask the subject
to compare the size of portions eaten with food models or photographs so that
they can make a better estimate of the quantities eaten. Ways of improving
quantity estimates with non-weighed record are shown in Box 12.3.

Attempts have been made to collect records by lending the respondent a camera
and asking them to take a photograph of each meal and snack eaten. Portion
weights can then be estimated more accurately by examining the photographs.

Food accounting

Food accounting methods estimate consumption indirectly by recording what
foods are purchased or removed for consumption from the household store

Box 12.3

Improving estimates of portion size in food diaries or 24-hour recall

Food replicas, pictures, photographs and real samples can all be used to help respondents quantify amounts of foods eaten. Most studies suggest that the use of food models improves the validity of reported intakes. However, they need to be used with care. An inappropriate size of model can bias results. Also the number of foods that can be represented by one set of models will be limited.

Food replicas and portion size models
Food replicas are three dimensional models made to represent specific foods. Portion models represent sizes of portions rather than specific foods and thus smaller sets can be used. Models can be made of many materials including rice set in wax, papier-mâché, wood, polystyrene and plastic. Bowls, spoons, graduated cups and glasses are also useful. Each model shape should have a graduated range of sizes including both smaller and larger than the usual portion size so as to reduce the likelihood of biasing reported consumption.

Photographs, pictures and drawings
Photographs and drawings have distinct advantages over food models. They are easier to produce locally and easy to carry about. Since they represent actual foods, they are easier to use to judge portion sizes.

Weighing of like-sized portions
In some circumstances it may be possible to obtain and weigh a similar portion to that eaten. Where food was obtained from a commercial outlet (e.g. a bag of chips) it is possible to buy a similar portion for weighing. If the subject can describe the shape and size of a portion of the food you can prepare and weigh a similar sized portion.

A detailed list of visual aids used for 24-hour recalls can be found in Cameron M. E. and Von Staveren W. E. (1988) *Manual on methodology for food consumption studies*. Oxford University Press, Oxford.

(larder, fridge, freezer etc). This enables foods taken for consumption to be accurately quantified with virtually no interference with the usual eating pattern. Unfortunately it is difficult to estimate how much of this food removed from store is not consumed. For foods which have to be cooked and prepared (potatoes, vegetables, untrimmed meats, etc.), the preparation and cooking losses are difficult to estimate. There will also be serving waste and plate waste.

The unit of food accounting is usually the household rather than the individual (all members of household consume food from same stores) so that food accounting methods generally estimate consumption by households rather than by individuals. If assumptions are made about how the food is distributed among household members then individual consumption can be crudely estimated from household consumption. The chief use of food accounting methods is as an independent check on other methods (criterion validation).

The National Food Survey is a special example of a survey using food accounting methods and is described at the end of this chapter.

Observation

In theory the ideal way to estimate actual food consumption would be to weigh everything unobtrusively before a person ate it and then to weigh any left overs. This would avoid the interference with usual eating habits caused by weighed inventory and food diary methods while giving very accurate data on quantities consumed. Of course it is usually impracticable to collect data in this way but in certain institutions where all the food is provided by one source it may be possible to collect weighed inventory data by observation. Where portion size is tightly controlled fairly accurate estimates of amount served can be made without weighing. It may not be too difficult to record what individual patients staying in a hospital ward or residential home eat all day or what a group of schoolchildren eat for lunch in the school canteen. This approach has been used successfully in military bases, college dormitories and communal homes in the USA.

Which method to use?

The final choice of method will depend on the aims of the study, the size of the sample, the accuracy and response rates required, the abilities and willingness to co-operate of participants and the resources available. The main advantages and disadvantages of each method are summarised in Table 12.1. Generally, the more accurate the method, the more expensive it will be to perform and the greater the risk of a low response rate because of the high degree of co-operation required from subjects.

The choice of method must depend on the purpose for which you are collecting the data. You will have to make a basic decision as to whether you want very detailed information on food consumption of relatively few people over a short period of time or whether you want less detailed information on a larger number of people. The food frequency questionnaire (Chapter 11) is probably the only practical method for studying very large numbers of people.

Table 12.1 Comparison of methods

	Food frequency questionnaire	24-hour recall	Diet diary	Weighed inventory
Type	General habit retrospective recall	Specified time retrospective recall	Specified time prospective as eaten	Specified time prospective as eaten
Time focus	Long term	Very short term	Short term	Short term
Interference with usual eating	Nil	Nil	High	Very high
Estimate of food quantity	Poor	Poor	Poor to fair	Good
Recall error	Large	Large	Small	Small
Difficulty for subject	Low	Low	Medium	High
Response rate	High	High	Fairly low	Low
Fieldworker skill needed	Low	High	Fairly high	High
Expense	Low	Medium	Medium	High

How many and which days?

When collecting diet records using either the weighed inventory or the food diary method one has to decide how long to continue. Usually seven days is the maximum length of time over which individuals can be expected to keep accurate records. However, inter-individual and intra-individual variations in nutrient intake can be large and various estimates have been made as to the number of days required for various nutrients (Box 12.4).

In practice seven days is the more usual time over which to collect records although some surveys have collected records for three or four days. Eating patterns may vary greatly at weekends and so at least one weekend day should be included in the survey period.

Box 12.4

How many days to collect?

There are very few data on variation in FOODS consumed over short periods of time but there have been several studies on variation in NUTRIENTS consumed over short periods of time. The number of days study required to estimate 'usual' consumption depends on the variation between days. (If all days were the same, one day's study would be adequate.)

The table below shows the numbers of days study required to be 95% confident that 80% of a population are appropriately classified into top, middle and bottom thirds of intake (tertiles). The figures are based on a population eating a typical British diet in the late 1970s.

NUTRIENT	MEN	WOMEN
Energy	5	4
Fat	9	6
Protein	5	5
Carbohydrate	3	2
Sugar	2	3
Fibre	10	5
Vitamin A	46	64
Vitamin C	6	6
Calcium	4	4
Iron	12	19
Fat as a % energy	18	7

Source:
James W. T., Bingham S. A. & Cole T. J. (1981). *Nutrition & Cancer 2*, 203-212.

How much time is needed to do a dietary survey?

Studies of food consumption are time consuming, whatever method is used. The time on a dietary study can be divided into two areas, the field work and the office work. The office work takes considerably more time than the field work. A breakdown of the time to be spent on various tasks is shown in Box 12.5.

Box 12.5

Time needed for a dietary survey

Field work
The field work can be roughly divided into four parts:

1   Recruitment of subjects
When recruiting a sample drawn from an electoral register or a GP's register, a great deal of time can be spent contacting the people selected, explaining the nature of the survey and persuading them to take part.
When the subjects come from a specific group, such as a school or club, recruiting may be much quicker once the approval and support of the head teacher or club leader has been obtained.

2   Interview time – i.e. the time spent with a subject
If a recall or diet history method is being used usually only one interview is required. A detailed diet history can take anything up to two hours to collect. For the collection of a food record by weighing or 'household' measures a minimum of three visits will be required. The first visit instructs the subject on the method. A second visit shortly after commencement of record keeping should check the subject has understood the instructions and a final visit goes through the completed record checking for inconsistency, clarifying entries, checking brands and recipes, etc. Interviews can vary from 15 minutes for quick check-up visits to an hour for first and final visits. In practice usually more than three visits will be required during a seven-day record. It is worth visiting subjects at least every other day and in some cases every day to maintain their motivation and co-operation.

3   'Friendly' time
This is the time spent 'socialising' with the subject. It can be considerable often taking more time than the interview. Most projects find this time increases as the record progresses. It is very important in maintaining subject motivation to participate conscientiously.

4   Travel time
Travel can take up a considerable part of the field work time. It includes abortive visits when subjects may be out despite prior arrangement. Even when visits are confined within a town or restricted geographical area, travel time can account for as much time as the interview.

Continued opposite

Box 12.5 (Continued)

Office work

1 Coding
Once records have been collected they will need to be coded for computing nutrient intakes. If every food item has been weighed and can be easily coded into food represented on the food composition tables this can be relatively straightforward. It takes longer to interpret portions recorded in household weights or by verbal description. It also takes much longer to code recipes not made up as standard cooked dishes.

2 Back-up work
This back-up work is needed to interpret and code diet records. It includes obtaining manufacturers' information on commercially prepared dishes, getting duplicate weights for unweighed food items, dissecting convenience and take-away meals and carrying out experimental cookery.

3 Preparing data for analysis
Data has to be entered for computer processing. It then has to be checked for coding and entry errors.

4 Analysis
The nutrient and other calculations have to be run. Outputs have to be summarised and analysed. This is a major task which may take as long as all the data collection and preparation.

One full-time fully trained fieldworker in an established dietary survey team could probably collect three seven-day weighed records in a week. For less experienced teams it is probably more realistic to expect each full-time worker to collect only two seven-day records. Fieldwork time will obviously depend on the number and lengths of interviews needed and where interviews will be conducted.

The staff needed

It is essential to obtain the services of a nutritionist or dietician for help with the design of the data collection, to train field staff or interviewers and to oversee coding and back-up work. You may be able to get this help from your local dietetic department or it may be possible to employ a freelance dietician on a short-term contract.

It is not necessary to employ fully trained dieticians or people with 'nutritional' backgrounds for the field work. Anyone who is alert and has a pleasant manner with people can be trained in a relatively short time to collect the dietary records. The key to success is to allow enough time for staff training and then make sure that the work of the fieldworkers is properly supervised and checked by the nutritionist or dietician (Box 12.6).

Box 12.6

Selection and training of fieldworkers for dietary surveys

Selection of interviewers
1   Must be alert, conscientious (and preferably a little obsessive!).
2   Must get on well with people and be persuasive.
3   No dietetic or nutritional experience needed.

Interviewer training
Interviewer training should cover the following aspects.
1   The purpose of the survey.
2   Detailed instructions on the collection of survey data.
3   Interview techniques.
4   Information on local foods, cooking techniques, etc.

Allow about one day for initial training of interviewers. They are then able to start data collection but will need careful supervision and checking.

Where to collect the data

Subjects can be visited in their own homes, or they can be asked to attend hospital or a local clinic where they can be interviewed. They can be interviewed over the phone or asked to return replies through the post. Each of these approaches has strengths and drawbacks. You have to choose the method best suited to your requirements.

Interviews in the home

This is the 'Rolls-Royce' approach. It is very convenient for the subject and it is easy to check replies but it means that a great deal of money and fieldworkers' time and money have to be used on travel.

The greater convenience for the subjects should improve response rate. The subject should be more relaxed and hence find it easier to recall food items.

Food items and brand labels can be shown to the interviewer along with usual household measures.

Apart from the large amount of time spent on travel there are other disadvantages to home interviewing. There may be interruptions from other members of the household. If it is not possible to interview the subject alone, other household members may influence the answers given, introducing bias.

It is also necessary to consider the safety of the interviewer and some sensible precautions are suggested in Box 12.7.

Less time is spent in travelling if data are being collected from several members of the same household or from people living very close together.

Box 12.7

Interviewer safety

If interviews are to be conducted in people's homes, it is important to consider the safety of the interviewer. Some simple ground rules should be followed.

1 Always make sure someone knows the address of the person being visited and how long the visit is expected to last. If this is not possible try to work in pairs.
2 Have identity cards, preferably with a photograph on them.
3 Only visit during daylight or if this is not possible don't visit after 9 p.m.
4 Be sensible: don't carry much money. Leave a situation if you feel unsafe.
5 If you are conducting a large survey, it is probably a good idea to notify the local police.

Remember many of your subjects may be nervous about you and reluctant to allow someone they do not know into their homes. Be sensitive to their needs for security.

Interviews in hospitals or clinics

Interviews that are held in hospital, clinic or local health centre are more convenient for the survey team, but less convenient for the subject. If subjects are already attending a clinic for another purpose it is easy to interview them during this appointment. If they are asked to attend just for the interview you will get a lower response rate.

Other disadvantages of interviews outside the home are that the subject may not be at ease, and it is not possible to check food packets and household portion sizes. On the other hand you may be able to use a larger set of portion models than you can reasonably take on home visits.

Can data be collected by telephone?

Telephone interviews can save considerably on travel time provided the subject has a phone. However, it is difficult to convey amounts of foods eaten by purely verbal description. Hence telephone interviews are more suitable for collecting food frequency information. Telephone interviews may be very useful for checking points on completed records or as a follow up to a face to face interview.

Could it be done by mail?

Food frequency questionnaires are the only method for which it is common to use the post. However, several surveys have asked people to complete 24-hour recalls and return the result by post and some have asked for 3-, 4- or even 7-day diet diaries through the post. If the subjects are able to compile reliable records in this way, then collecting data through the post saves a great deal of time and makes it possible to obtain data from many more people.

The problem with postal 24-hour recalls or diet diaries is that there is less opportunity to prompt the subject's memory or to help them describe food quantities. An attempt can be made to fill in missing information by phoning the subjects but there is little opportunity to clarify points in the record which are unclear or to seek additional details on foods. There must therefore be considerable doubt as to whether 24-hour recalls or diet diaries collected through the post without prior training can be used for any purpose more than estimating food consumption frequencies. Postal extensions to studies begun with face to face data collection may be effective.

Can the computer do dietary interviews?

Dietary information can be collected using specifically designed computer programs which ask the subject a series of questions about their dietary patterns and what food they have recently eaten. Programs have now been devised which can probe dietary patterns quite effectively. Use of a computer in this way saves interviewer time and many subjects find it easier to communicate frankly with a machine than a person. (Machines do not pass judgement or raise their eyebrows when you admit to drinking a bottle of whisky each night.) There is probably considerable scope for this approach in situations such as clinics and outpatient departments. However, a dietician and a programmer probably will

Box 12.8

The National Food Survey

The National Food Survey (NFS) is conducted annually for the Ministry of Agriculture, Fisheries and Food. Data are collected throughout the year from a random sample of approximately 7,000 private households throughout Great Britain.

Each survey household records amounts of all food intended for human consumption entering the home during the survey period of seven days. Information is also collected on the number of meals eaten outside the home but not on the composition of those meals. Soft drinks bought into the household are recorded but not at present included in the main analyses. Sweets, chocolates, alcoholic drinks and foods consumed outside the home are not covered in the survey. It is generally accepted that the NFS underestimates the quantities of snack foods eaten.

Information provided by the National Food Survey
The results of the NFS are now published as an annual report a year after the survey is completed under the title 'Household Food Consumption and Expenditure'. Copies can be found in academic libraries or can be purchased from any HMSO bookshop. (The report for 1989, published in 1990, cost £19.75.)

The report includes various analyses of trends in food and nutrient consumption and expenditure, and a useful set of supplementary tables comparing the nutritional value of household foods by income group, family size and region.

Earlier reports of the National Food Survey contained more detailed tables on consumption. The NFS can still supply these extra analyses if requested but charge commercial fees for this service. Further information can be obtained from National Food Survey Branch, Ministry of Agriculture, Fisheries and Food, Room 419, West Block, Whitehall Place, London SW1A 2HM.

have to devote several hundred hours to programming if you have to develop a new system.

Conducting an interview

People are more likely to respond well to the interview if the interviewer has a friendly manner. Interviews should begin by putting the subject at ease and with a brief explanatory introduction. The interviewer should stress the importance

185

of giving truthful answers. Sufficient time must be allowed for the respondent to answer questions and excessive prompting must be avoided. It is important to ask neutral questions, and not to show approval or disapproval of any answers given.

The National Food Survey

The main source of information on the diet of the United Kingdom population is the National Food Survey (NFS). The great strength of the NFS is that it is based on a large and fairly representative sample.

Its main disadvantages are that it collects information on households not individuals and largely excludes foods eaten outside the home. The published reports use rather broad food groupings.

The NFS collects information on basic ingredients, rather than foods consumed. For example if the household consumes home cooked chips, the NFS reports the fat and the potatoes as separate items. This makes no overall difference to the total fat or energy content of the diet, but does make a difference to the type of information obtained about particular prepared items. Further information on the NFS is given in Box 12.8.

Further reading

General

Cameron M. E. & Van Staveren W. A. (1988).
  Manual on Methodology for Food Consumption Studies. Oxford University Press, Oxford.
James W. P. T., Bingham S. A. & Cole T. J. (1981). 'Epidemiological assessment of dietary intake.'
  Nutrition & Cancer 2, 203-212.
Marr J. W. (1971). 'Individual dietary surveys: purposes and methods.'
  World Review of Nutrition and Dietetics 13, 105-164.

The photographic method

Elwood P. C. & Bird G. (1983). 'A photographic method of diet evaluation.'
  Human Nutrition: Applied Nutrition 37A, 474-477.
Fehily A. M & Bird G. (1984). 'The dietary intakes of women in Caerphilly, South Wales. A weighed and a photographic method compared.'
  Human Nutrition: Applied Nutrition 40A, 300-307.

Recall method

Dwyer J. T., Krall E. A. & Coleman K. A. (1987). 'The problem of memory in nutritional epidemiological research.'
Journal of American Dietetic Association 87, 1509-1512.

The dietary history method

Burke B. S. (1947). 'The dietary history as a tool in research.'
Journal of American Dietetic Association 23, 1041-1046. (This paper is frequently cited but those who cite it rarely use the methods described in it.)

Validity of methods

Klesges R. C., Hansom C. L., Eck L. H. & Durff A. C. (1988). 'Accuracy of self-reports of food intake in obese and normal weight individuals.'
American Journal of Clinical Nutrition 48, 1252-1256.

Mahalko J. R., Johnson L. K., Gallagher S. K. & Milne D. B. (1985). 'Comparison of dietary histories and seven-day food records in a nutritional assessment of older adults.'
American Journal of Clinical Nutrition 42, 542-553.

Logistics of dietary surveys

Black A. E. (1988). Chap. 13 'Economic appraisal of various study designs and methods.' In Cameron M. E. & Van Staveren W. A. (see above).

Black A. E. (1982). 'The logistics of dietary surveys.'
Human Nutrition: Applied Nutrition 36A, 85-94.

Use of computers for interviewing

Slack W., Porter D., Witschi J., Sullivan M., Buxbaum R. & Stare J. (1976). 'Dietary interviewing by computer.'
Journal of American Dietetic Association 69, 514-517.

Levine J. A., Madden A. M. & Morgan M. Y. (1987). 'Validation of a computer-based system for assessing dietary intake.'
British Medical Journal 295, 369-372.

How many days to record

Marr J. W. & Heady J. A. (1986). 'Within and between person variation in dietary surveys: Number of days needed to classify individuals.'
Human Nutrition: Applied Nutrition 40A, 347-364.

Van Staveren W. A., Burema J., Deurenberg P. & Katan M. B. (1988). 'Weak associations in nutrition epidemiology: The importance of replication of observations on individuals.'
International Journal of Epidemiology 17, 964-969.

The National Food Survey

Derry B. J. & Buss D. H. (1984). 'The British National Food Survey as a major epidemiological resource.'
British Medical Journal 288, 765-767.

13 · Estimating nutrient intake

Summary

Consumption may be described either in terms of food or terms of nutrients. The most appropriate way of expressing consumption data will depend on the purpose for which it is to be used.

Nutrient intake can be estimated with data from weighed inventory, food diary and 24-hour recall. The use of food composition tables introduce major additional errors. Very crude estimates of nutrient intake can also be made from food frequency questionnaires. When designing a questionnaire intended to estimate nutrient intake you must include those foods which are major sources of those nutrients in which you are interested. The major food sources of energy, fat, fibre, iron, calcium and vitamin C are described.

Foods or nutrients?

We can describe daily intakes in terms of food (meat, potatoes, fruit etc.) or in terms of nutrients (calories, fats, starch, fibre, calcium, iron, vitamin C, riboflavin and so on). Each approach has its advantages and disadvantages.

If we describe consumption in food terms then it is relatively easy for all to understand. Everyone knows what an orange is but people may have difficulty in understanding what is meant by riboflavin (or even by fat when a nutritionist is using the word). Healthier eating messages are likely to be given in food terms (e.g. eat more wholemeal bread) rather than in nutrient terms. Therefore when attempting to evaluate the direct impact of health promotion activities it may be more appropriate to express consumption in food terms.

On the other hand it is difficult to assess the nutritional significance of a list of quantities of the many different foods consumed by a person in a week. It is nutrients which are known to be important for health and not the foods from which they came. One gramme of vitamin C has the same effect on the body regardless of whether it came from oranges, potato crisps or the chemist's laboratory. We can only tell whether someone's nutrient intake is adequate or compare one person's nutrient intake with another's if we first convert the consumption information into nutrients.

When we convert food consumption data into nutrient intake we lose a great deal of information. A gramme of fibre from wholemeal bread is not identical to a gramme of fibre obtained from green vegetables and a gramme of saturated fat from beef is not identical to a gramme of saturated fat from lamb.

Food consumption patterns and nutrient intake

We have to calculate nutrient intake from all food sources to see whether a shift in consumption of an individual food is associated with changes in the total intake of any nutrient since consumption of other foods may also change. Food frequency data (how often people consume different foods) can be useful for monitoring shifts in eating patterns and compliance with healthier eating advice but are not a totally reliable guide to nutrient intakes (Figure 13.1). For example, the consumption of reduced fat milks has increased over the past years but the percent of energy from fat in the UK diet has remained static.

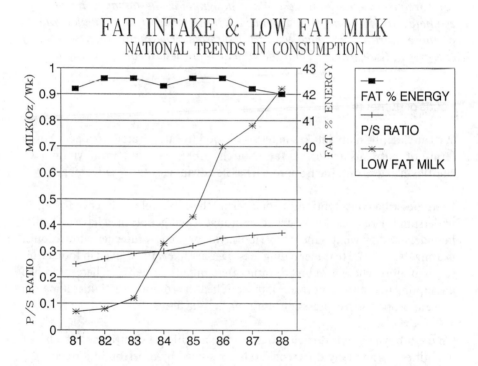

FAT INTAKE & LOW FAT MILK
NATIONAL TRENDS IN CONSUMPTION

Figure 13.1   Trends in consumption of skimmed milks, total fat and P:S ratio

Note that total fat consumption remains virtually unchanged while consumption of skimmed milks rises.

Data taken from NFS.

Calculating nutrient intake from specified time methods data

Weighed inventory studies provide information on what foods and what quantities of them are eaten throughout the day. It is relatively easy to convert this data into nutrient data by multiplying the weight of each food consumed by the amount of nutrient in that food (provided we know its nutrient content).

$$\text{Nutrient Consumed} = \frac{\text{Weight of food}}{100} \times \text{nutrient per 100 gramme of food}$$

Data from diet diary studies or 24-hour recall can similarly be converted into estimates of nutrient intake using the estimated weight of each food consumed.

However, it is totally impracticable to analyse chemically the nutrient content of duplicate samples of the foods eaten. Hence the quantity of nutrient per 100 gramme of food is obtained from food composition tables. The food tables most widely used in the UK are McCance and Widdowson (4th edition) which contain data on some 850 different foods and 27 different nutrients plus less complete data on 30 other nutrients. The new UK food tables (published as supplement to McCance and Widdowson) contain data on many more foods and 16 other nutrients. A revised and expanded 5th edition has just been published.

Food table errors

These sorts of calculations can easily produce a spurious impression of accuracy and it is important to realise that converting food intake data into nutrient intake data using food composition tables introduces a major additional source of error.

The values given in food tables are intended to be representative for each food. Yet of course two samples of the same food from different sources at different times are most unlikely to be chemically identical. The nutrient content of the apple or cake eaten by a respondent can differ substantially from the nutrient content for that food which is listed in the food tables. Where a food has been cooked the errors are likely to be even larger since the conditions in which it was prepared, cooked and served can all affect the nutrient content. The nutrient content of the boiled potatoes given in the food tables is unlikely to be the same as that of the boiled potatoes eaten by someone on any particular occasion.

The errors are larger for some nutrients than for others. Water content of foods is very variable as is content of vitamin C and other water soluble vitamins, minerals and fatty acids. For some nutrients the food tables are incomplete and unless special care is taken (especially with computerised food tables) foods for which a particular nutrient content is not known may be treated as containing none of that nutrient.

Approximate coding of foods is a further source of error. Although the food tables contain a wide variety of foods there will be many foods which are not listed in the food tables. The various ways of coding these foods are shown in Box 13.1 but all introduce further errors.

The errors arising from conversion of food intake into nutrient intake may often be greater than the errors due to inaccurate estimation of food quantity.

Box 13.1

Methods of coding foods not included in food tables

1 Code to nearest approximation in food tables
    e.g. Commercial apple pie   Code as jam tart
           Courgette   Code as marrow

2 Code to constituent parts
    e.g. Jaffa Cake   Code as chocolate + jam + sponge

3 Create new code calculated from ingredients and recipe
    e.g. Meat and vegetable stew
    Add nutrient contents of ingredients and correct for nutrient losses during cooking to estimate nutrient content of final dish.

Estimation of nutrient intake from food frequency questionnaires

Because of the practical difficulty of obtaining weighed inventories, diet diaries or 24-hour recalls many attempts have been made to estimate nutrient intake using data from food frequency questionnaires. The design of a questionnaire for this purpose poses many extra difficulties. The two main issues are whether we can obtain useful information on portion size (discussed in Chapter 11) and which foods we should ask about.

The design of the questionnaire depends on what we are trying to find out. A questionnaire intended to throw light on sources of vitamin C in the diet would be totally inappropriate for studying the percentage of energy derived from fat.

The ways in which nutrient intake might be estimated from data obtained by use of a food frequency questionnaire are shown in Box 13.2. Lack of adequate information on portion size is a major weakness in these estimates and some question whether food frequency data should be used in this way at all. The errors can be somewhat reduced if it is possible to collect information on portion size for a few foods where this is a major source of variability. If estimates of nutrient intake are derived from food frequency data, it is absolutely essential that the methods of estimation should be validated on the populations in which they are to be used.

Box 13.2

Estimation of nutrient intake from food frequency questionnaires

It is important to realise that any estimate of nutrient intake based on food frequency questionnaires will be very crude because:

1 There is no reliable measure of quantity consumed.
2 Foods of different composition are likely to be combined into single food groups.
3 Some foods may not be mentioned on the questionnaire.

There are two methods of producing formulae for the conversion of food frequency data to nutrient intake data:

      i)   Analogy with weighed intake data

and ii) Pragmatic derivation of weightings. (Optimisation)

Analogy with weighed intake data
The amount of nutrient derived from a particular food (N) is given by:

$$N = F \times P \times C$$

Where F is the frequency with which the food is consumed by the respondent.
          P is the average portion size in the population.
          C is the nutrient content of unit weight of the food.

P and C are constants so the total nutrient intake (TN) becomes:

$$TN = (F_1 \times W_1) + (F_2 \times W_2) + (F_3 \times W_3)\dots\dots\dots\dots\dots\dots + (F_n \times W_n) + R$$

Where F_1, F_2, F_3 are the frequencies with which each food is consumed.
          W_1, W_2, W_3 are corresponding weightings for each food derived from average portion size and average nutrient contents.
          R is term for nutrient derived from foods not covered in questionnaire.

Appropriate weightings for each food are estimated by consideration of mixture of foods in each food group, nutrient composition of those foods and observations of usual portion size for those foods. An example of this approach is the 'Caerphilly' questionnaire (Yarnell *et al.* (1983) *Human Nutrition: Applied Nutrition 37A*, 103-112).

Continued overleaf

Box 13.2 (Continued)

Pragmatic derivation of weightings (Optimisation)
This method also produces a formula for total nutrient intake (TN) of the type:

$$TN = (F_1 \times W_1) + (F_2 \times W_2) + (F_3 \times W_3) \dotfill + (F_n \times W_n) + K$$

Where F_1, F_2, F_3 are the frequencies with which each food is consumed.
W_1, W_2, W_3 are corresponding weightings.
K is a constant.

However, the method by which the weightings are derived is totally different. The food frequency data for a group of individuals is compared with nutrient intake data from the same individuals derived from some other method (usually weighed inventory or 24-hour recall). The values of W_1, W_2, W_3 etc. and K are then derived by multiple regression or some similar technique.

This method makes no assumption about the rationale for each weighting but merely optimises the fit between the predicted and actual nutrient intake. It is therefore possible for foods to have negative weightings.

For example frequency of consumption of low fat spreads may have a negative weighting for prediction of fat intake because people who eat this food frequently tend to have low fat intakes. Similarly foods may contribute to the prediction of intake of nutrients which they do not contain. For example frequency of consumption of skimmed milk may contribute to the prediction of fibre intake because people who drink skimmed milk tend to eat a lot of fibre-rich foods.

Often there is no apparent nutritional explanation for a term in a prediction formula produced by the pragmatic method. Many workers feel uncomfortable with terms whose inclusion cannot be rationalised and exclude them from the final formulae.

Formulae to predict nutrient intakes should always be validated on a different data set from that used to produce them.

An example of a pragmatically produced formula is that of Hankin J. H. *et al.* (1968) *American Journal of Epidemiology 87*, 285-298.

Which foods to ask about

It is not obvious which foods should be included when you are interested in intake of a particular nutrient. It might seem reasonable to find out which foods are rich in the nutrients of interest to you (see Table 13.1) and then to ask questions about those foods.

Table 13.1　Foods rich in certain nutrients

Note that this list is NOT a basis for selecting foods for inclusion in a food frequency questionnaire intended to estimate consumption of these nutrients.

Fat
Foods containing more than 35 g fat/100 g
Cream cheese, bacon, butter, margarine, nuts
Foods containing more than 20 g fat/100 g
Sausage, roast lamb, roast pork, black pudding, potato crisps, chocolate cheesecake.

Fibre
Foods containing more than 12 g fibre/100 g
All bran, whole wheat breakfast cereals, dried beans (cooked), dried fruit, almonds and some nuts.
Foods containing more than 8 g fibre/100 g
Wholemeal bread, cornflakes, crispbread, lentils, potato crisps, peanuts and some nuts.

Vitamin C
Foods containing more than 60 mg Vit C/100 g
Green peppers, cauliflowers, spinach, watercress, blackcurrants, strawberries.
Foods containing more than 30 mg Vit C/100 g
Brussel sprouts, grapefruit, gooseberries, oranges, lemon juice, orange juice.

However, the importance of a food as a dietary source of any nutrient depends not only on how much of the nutrient it contains but also on how much of the food is eaten. Therefore a food which has a high content of a particular nutrient will only be a major source of that nutrient in the diet of the population if it is eaten in reasonable quantities. For example, offals such as liver are considered a food source of iron but only contribute 2.8% of the iron in the current UK diet because little is eaten. In fact the top four sources of iron in the current UK diet are white bread and flour (14.9%), breakfast cereal (8.8%), potatoes (6.6%) and wholemeal bread (4.4%).

The first step in designing a questionnaire should therefore be to examine the main sources of the nutrients of interest in the population under study. For populations in the UK the National Food Survey can be consulted to find the likely main sources. Further useful data on nutrient sources in English men derived from another study have been published (Box 13.3).

Remember that if your interests are in a particular sub-group of the population (e.g. Vegans, Asians, pregnant or lactating women, children, men in a particular age band, people relying on state benefit, etc.) their nutrient sources may well be different from those of the total population so that data from generalised surveys such as the National Food Survey would not be an appropriate guide to their nutrient sources.

Food sources of selected nutrients

This section considers which foods need to be included when designing questionnaires to study intakes of selected nutrients.

1   Energy

Forty percent of the UK energy intake comes from dairy products, meat and fats (Fig 13.2). Within these broad food groupings, individual foods contribute small but significant amounts of energy, for example, cheese contributes 2.7% of total energy, fish 1.3% and eggs 1.3%. Within the fruit and vegetable group potatoes contribute 3.7% of total energy, other vegetables 4.3% and fruit and fruit juices 3.0%. Breakfast cereals contribute 2.6% of total energy. Cakes, biscuits and pastries contribute 6.7% total energy and confectionery items 5.9%.

Data from another source (Box 13.3) suggests that as few as 37 food items account for 90% of the energy in the diet. It should be noted that foods with the highest energy contents are not necessarily major sources of energy in the diet overall.

2   Fat

The major sources of fat in the UK diet are spreading and cooking fats, meat and meat products and dairy foods (Fig 13.2). These three food groups account for just over three-quarters of the UK fat intake. Within these groups certain foods make a significant contribution, for example, cheese contributes 6% of

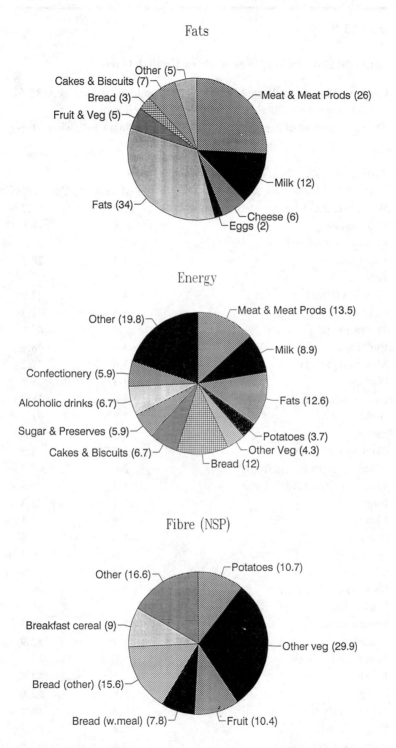

Figure 13.2 Food sources of nutrients in UK diet

Data taken from NFS 1985.

Box 13.3

Nutrient sources in survey of three English towns

Cade and Margetts collected data from 2340 middle-aged subjects (35-54 years) living in three English towns using 24-hour diet diaries. The main sources of energy fat and fibre are given in the following tables:

TABLE A   Sources of energy in the diet

Food	% of total	Cumulative %
White bread and flour	11.7	11.7
Milk – whole	6.9	18.6
Potatoes – not fried	4.8	23.4
Sugar (table)	4.8	28.2
Beer	4.5	32.7
Potatoes (fried)	4.3	37.0
Cakes	4.3	41.3
Margarine (all)	3.7	45.0
Puddings	3.6	48.6
Meat and pastry dishes	3.6	52.2
Biscuits	3.3	55.5
Cheese – high fat	3.0	58.5
Butter	2.7	61.2
Bacon	2.3	63.5
Cooked meat dishes	2.0	65.5
Wholemeal bread and flour	2.0	67.5
Breakfast cereal (all)	1.9	69.4
Eggs	1.9	71.3
Fish	1.8	73.1
Sausages	1.8	74.9
Beef	1.6	76.5
Chicken	1.4	77.9
Sweets and chocolate	1.4	79.3
Pork	1.3	80.6
Brown bread	1.2	81.8
Squash and soft drinks	1.1	82.9
Sauces and pickles	1.0	83.9
Lamb	0.9	84.8
Crisps	0.8	85.6
Wine and sherry	0.8	86.4
Sweet spreads	0.8	87.2
Cheese and egg dishes	0.6	87.8
Canned meats	0.6	88.4

Continued opposite

Box 13.3 (Continued)

Food	% of total	Cumulative %
Tea and coffee	0.5	88.9
Apples	0.5	89.4
Milk – skimmed	0.5	89.9
Crackers, crispbread	0.5	90.4

TABLE B   Sources of fat in the diet

Food	% of total	Cumulative %
Milk – whole	9.6	9.6
Margarine (not PUFA)	7.4	17.0
Butter	7.1	24.1
Cheese – high fat	5.9	30.0
Meat and pastry dishes	5.6	35.6
Potatoes – fried	4.6	40.2
Cakes	4.4	44.6
Puddings	3.9	48.5
Bacon	3.9	52.4
White bread and flour	3.7	56.1
Biscuits	3.7	59.8
Eggs	3.7	63.5
Sausages	3.0	66.5
Cooked meat dishes	2.8	69.3
PUFA margarine	2.4	71.7
Potatoes – not fried	2.2	73.9
Beef	2.1	76.0
Pork	2.0	78.0
Sauces and pickles	1.6	79.6
Lamb	1.6	81.2
Chicken	1.5	82.7
Sweets and chocolate	1.4	84.1
Crisps	1.4	85.5
White fish – fried	1.1	86.6
Canned meat	1.1	87.7
Fish – oily	1.0	88.7
Cheese and egg dishes	1.0	89.7
Low fat spread	0.6	90.3

TABLE C   Sources of total dietary fibre in the diet

Food	% of total	Cumulative %
White bread and flour	14.6	14.6
Whole meal bread and flour	9.8	24.4
Potatoes – not fried	8.6	33.0
Breakfast cereal	8.2	41.2

Continued overleaf

Box 13.3 (Continued)

Food	% of total	Cumulative %
Peas	7.5	48.7
Potatoes – fried	6.0	54.7
Baked beans	4.4	59.1
Brown bread	3.1	62.2
Cakes	2.8	65.0
Biscuits	2.7	67.7
Apples	2.4	70.1
Carrots	2.4	72.5
Crisps	2.2	74.7
Puddings	2.1	76.8
Tomato	2.0	78.8
Meat and pastry dishes	1.6	80.4
Cooked meat dishes	1.2	81.6
Cabbage	1.2	82.8
Brussels sprouts	1.2	84.0
Oranges	1.0	85.0
Crackers, crispbread	0.9	85.9
Banana	0.9	86.8
Beans	0.8	87.6
Cauliflower	0.7	88.3
Onion	0.7	89.0
Pears	0.7	89.7
Peanuts	0.5	90.2

total fat intake. Fat with chips is included in cooking fats but data from another source (Box 13.3) suggests that these account for nearly 5% of fat intake.

By and large the major sources of fat are also the major sources of saturated fat. The major source of polyunsaturated fats are the polyunsaturated margarines and particular vegetable oils. Thus, if one is concerned with the type of fat consumed, it is important to ask about the type of margarines and oils used.

3 Fibre

The major food group sources of dietary fibre are shown in Figure 13.2. This figure groups all vegetables together but not all vegetables are equally important as fibre sources. In another study (Box 13.3) peas were found to contribute 7.5% and baked beans to contribute 4.4% of the fibre in the diet.

Qualitative information about the types of food eaten is particularly important in studies concerned with fibre intake. It is for example, essential to ask about the type of bread consumed as this is a better predictor of fibre intake than the total amount of bread consumed. Questions should also be asked about the type of breakfast cereal consumed since choosing high fibre cereals is a predictor of high intakes of fibre.

Dietary fibre is a complex mixture of substances chiefly derived from plant cell walls and you may want to know about the intakes of the different types of fibre rather than the total fibre intake. More information on the different types of fibre is given in Box 13.4.

Foods which ought to be included in a food frequency questionnaire concerned with energy, fat and fibre are shown in Table 13.2.

Table 13.2   Foods sources of energy, fat and fibre

% of total nutrient intake contributed by each food.

**** More than 20%, *** More than 10%, ** More than 5%, * More than 2%, – Negligible, 0 None

	Energy	Fat	Fibre
Meat and meat products	***	****	–
Fats (butter, margarine etc.)	***	****	0
Bread	***	*	****
Milk	**	***	0
Cakes and biscuits	**	**	*
Alcoholic drinks	**	0	0
Confectionery	**	*	–
Sugar & jam	**	0	–
Potatoes	**	*	***
Other vegetables	*	–	****
Fruit & fruit juice	*	–	***
Cheese	*	**	0
Breakfast cereals	*	–	**
Other foods	10%	8%	17%

---

4   Iron and Calcium

Cereals contribute 46% of iron in the UK diet, this coming from bread and flour (24.8%), cakes, pastries and biscuits (6.3%), breakfast cereals (11.9%), meat contributes 18.2%, of the iron (liver contributes 1.7%), vegetables 16.8% (potatoes account for 4.2%), and fruit 4.1%, milk and fish contribute 2.6% and 2% respectively.

Box 13.4

What is fibre?

Dietary fibre has been defined as matter of plant origin (mostly cell walls) which is incompletely digested by the human gut. Chemically most but not all dietary fibres are a kind of complex carbohydrate called polysaccharides. Some dietary fibres are hard, tough and insoluble in water while others are soft, viscous and soluble in water.

Components of dietary fibre
  Polysaccharides
  Cellulose
  Hemicellulose
  Pectic substances
  Mucilages
  Gums
  Algal polysaccharides
  Lignin (not a carbohydrate)

The analysis of fibre in foods is difficult and different methods give different fibre contents. One way of measuring fibre is to measure the non-starch polysaccharides (NSP). This is the method currently used for the National Food Survey which shows that the average UK diet contains approximately 13-14 g NSP.

Cereals, fruits and vegetables are rich sources of dietary fibre but the types of fibre in cereals and vegetables are different.

Further information is given in Royal College of Physicians (1980). *Medical aspects of dietary fibre*. Pitman Medical.

Iron from animal sources may be more available than iron from plant sources. It may therefore be important to distinguish iron from these two sources.

The National Food Survey suggests the main sources of calcium in the UK diet to be milk (providing 44.7%), cheese (13.3%) and bread and flour (18.5%).

5   Vitamin C

The main sources of Vitamin C in the UK diet are fruit juice (27.1%), fruit (19.8%), potatoes (13.6%), other vegetables (29.6%) and milk (4.8%). Soft drinks may also be a significant source of Vitamin C but are not included in this list since they are not adequately covered in the National Food Survey.

Further reading

Estimation of nutrient intake by questionnaire

Hankin J. H., Stallones R. A. and Messenger H. B. (1968). 'A short dietary method for epidemiologic studies.'
American Journal of Epidemiology 87, 285-298.

Yarnell J. W. G., Milbank J., Walker C. L., Fehily A. M. & Hayes T. *et al.* (1983). 'A short dietary questionnaire for use in epidemiological survey: Comparison with weighed dietary records.'
Human Nutrition: Applied Nutrition 37A, 103-122.

Gray G. E., Paganini-Hill A., Ross R. K. & Henderson B. E. (1984). 'Assessment of three brief methods of estimation of vitamin A and C intake for a prospective study of cancer.'
American Journal of Epidemiology 119, 581-590.

Willet W. C., Sampson L., Stampfer M. S. and five others (1985). 'Reproducibility and validity of a semi-quantitative food frequency questionnaire.'
American Journal of Public Health 122, 51-65.

Shepherd R. and Farleigh C. A. (1987). 'Salt intake assessment by questionnaire and urinary sodium excretion.'
Nutrition Research 7, 557-568.

Livingstone M. B. E., Prentice A. M., Strain J. J., and five others (1990). 'Accuracy of weighed records in studies of diet and health.'
British Medical Journal 300, 708-713.

Food sources of nutrient

Cade J. E. and Margetts B. M. (1988). 'Nutrient sources in the English diet: Quantitative data from three English towns.'
International Journal of Epidemiology 17, 844-848.

UK food tables

'McCance and Widdowson's'
The Composition of Foods (5th edition) 1991
Supplements to 4th edition
1st Supplement – 'Amino Acids and Fatty Acids'
2nd Supplement – 'Immigrant Foods'
3rd Supplement – 'Cereal and cereal products'
4th Supplement – 'Milk products and eggs'
5th Supplement – 'Vegetables, Herbs and Spices'
Obtainable from Royal Society of Chemistry, Sales and Promotion Department, Thomas Grabham House, Milton Road, Cambridge CB4 4WF.

14 · Measuring food consumption – trends in retail food sales and food purchase

by Mike Clapham and Neil J. G. Field

Summary

Food reaches the consumer through a supply chain stretching back to the original producer. Changes in consumer consumption are only possible if there are corresponding changes all down the food supply chain.

Consumer purchasing behaviour is affected by the availability of foods and the way in which it is marketed.

In order to understand how local consumers are changing their food buying patterns and what is influencing them information should be sought from local retail food outlets.

Information on national and regional trends can be sought from producers alliances, food processors and retail chains.

Sales in catering outlets can also be monitored to study the effects of healthier eating promotions.

How food reaches the consumer

When you research into retail food sales and the trends of consumption, it is helpful to look at the chain of supply and its links from the production of food through to the consumer (Figure 14.1). Unless the links fit and join together then the chain is ineffective. This is why when there is a smoothly operating chain of supply for a particular food it is difficult to introduce a 'healthier' alternative without first taking note of and adjusting to the needs of all the people making up the links in the chain. Changes in consumer demand for a product will affect all links in the chain. If production cannot rise to meet an increased consumer demand then the price is likely to rise.

Figure 14.1   The food supply chain

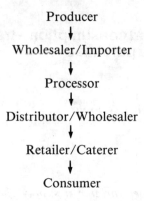

Producer
↓
Wholesaler/Importer
↓
Processor
↓
Distributor/Wholesaler
↓
Retailer/Caterer
↓
Consumer

The operation of the food supply chain can be illustrated with two examples.

Fish sales

Fish is an example of a product where increased demand in the face of restricted supply results in consumption being chiefly controlled by fluctuating prices. The natural supplies of fish are limited so that the producers cannot readily increase the supply entering the chain. The main effect of current efforts to persuade the consumer to buy more fish are likely to be rising prices as retailers and distributors compete to obtain the limited supplies. The scope for increasing consumption of fish is restricted by the operation of the food chain and limited supply.

Polyunsaturated oils

Polyunsaturated oil, by contrast, has been a success story with supply expanding to meet increased consumer demand. Originally there was little demand for polyunsaturated oils; lard was the main fat used for cooking and oil was generally difficult to find in the shops. The processors then developed an improved product. New sources of raw material and better refining methods produced a blandly flavoured oil. Labelling emphasising the polyunsaturate content gave the product a 'healthy' image. This message was supported in more general terms by the healthy eating movement (? health education). The improved oil was sold in attractive lightweight bottles. Advertising by the retailers and distributors vigorously stressed the selling points of the product, its newness, freshness, ease of use, safety and healthiness. The new product became a sales success competing with and displacing traditional lard-type hard fats. As the market has expanded, farmers throughout the world have increased their acreages of rape, sunflower, or ground nuts to meet the increased demand and supplement oils from the traditional olive and palm groves.

The case of polyunsaturated oil shows how all parts of the chain have had to pull together to get this 'new healthier' product to the consumer. The consumer had to be convinced that the oil was safe and easy to use and could then be motivated to purchase because of a growing concern for health. The supply end of the chain responded and a steady and continuing increase in consumption of polyunsaturated oils was seen throughout all the western world.

If the product had been too expensive in comparison with the hard fats only the wealthy or the health cranks would have bought. Because the supply increased to meet the consumer demand, price did not rise and the oil was sold at a price at which it became a competitive product and was widely used.

The decision of the consumer to buy is influenced by two things:
1   Availability
2   Marketing

Availability

The final link in the supply chain is usually the retailer. It is evidently true for any product that 'if it is not on the shelves, it cannot be bought'. Just a few years ago, supermarkets in less affluent neighbourhoods would not stock such 'healthy' items as wholemeal bread, skimmed milk and vegetable oils. This meant that these foods were not available to their customers and so were not bought. The shopkeepers explained the non-availability of these items by saying that they only carried a restricted number of lines and anyway their customers would not buy them. Of course customers did not buy articles which were not in the shop. Times have changed and those shopkeepers who took the risk of stocking the 'healthier' lines have found that once they were made available the customers would buy.

Marketing

The magic word marketing covers all the activities which encourage the customer to buy a food:
i   Packaging, labelling and brand names
ii   Advertising
iii   Coupons and special promotions
iv   Point of sale presentation
v   Pricing.

All of these influence the acceptability of the product by the consumer and thus increase the likelihood of sales of a food that proves palatable.

Gathering information from food sales outlets

The customer may purchase foods from institutional caterers, caterers, shops, markets, co-operatives, supermarkets or direct from producers (farm shops, quayside). Information on food sales from all of these outlets may be very helpful in showing trends in food purchase which may (or may not) be due to the operation of district food policies.

It is often said that it is very difficult to get sales information from privately run companies, but you never know what information you can get unless you ask. You may not even be sure what information you want from them but talking to companies and institutions can be very useful. They may give you the information which will help you see trends in food habits or other information which will be helpful in planning future health promotion. For example they may tell you of trends in sales of certain items (e.g. wholemeal bread sales have increased by 12% in the past year) or they may inform you of future promotions that they are planning which could tie in with your activities.

Go and look at local shops

The following story illustrates the need to visit local shops in order to understand what may influence food purchases by consumers in your district. A particular supermarket displayed its skimmed milk on pallets in the store. Once the milk had been sold, it could not be replaced during the busy periods because the fork lift truck was considered too dangerous for use when shoppers were in the store. Therefore, once the milk on the pallet was sold no more could be bought that day. This story demonstrates how a relatively simple factor can restrict consumption of a food and the problem could only be understood by visiting the point of sale. Before mounting a campaign to increase purchase of a particular food you must check that your retailers can respond.

There is no substitute for a walk about. Go and have a look. What is favourable, how much shelf space is given to certain food items and where is it displayed? Inform the local companies what you wish to do. You never know: they may wish to help you. In the case of national companies it is sometimes better to work with the local store manager than through head office.

The golden rules in seeking information from local sales outlets are:
  i   Always ask, you never know what you might get.
  ii Go and have a look at as many as possible.
      See both how the food is displayed and what the shoppers do.

Local monitoring of retail food sales

First of all chat-up and make friends with your local manager. This is not as difficult as you might at first think. Most managers these days are naturally very keen to be 'in' on the trends of consumption. They know about healthy eating and are often quite willing to co-operate with studies that show trends. At the simplest level (and thus most likely to be agreed by the manager) you could decide to choose a number of foods or, better still, brands of foods and monitor the changes in their sales over a period of time. Of course actual sales figures are commercially sensitive information but a comparison of sales by the manager could result in him being able to say 'over the last six months wholemeal bread sales increased by 12%'. See Box 14.1 for an example of this approach.

The way to proceed is choose your foods, choose your outlets, decide on the length of the study and the frequency of collecting the data. Convince the manager that it is a useful survey and that they will be given good feedback that could benefit the store. Then get on with it!

Box 14.1

Example of trend in local retail food sales

A number of supermarkets in Worcester were approached and asked to supply information on sales of selected food items over the period October 1984-October 1985. A campaign to promote healthier eating was mounted in the district in early 1985. The changes seen are in the direction advocated by the campaign. Could the campaign have contributed to the changes?

Food item	% Change
Brown breads including wholemeal	+ 170
White bread	+ 2
Lard	− 20
Butter	− 2
Polyunsaturated oil	+ 95
Polyunsaturated margarine	+ 45
Fat reduced cheese	+ 90
Skimmed/semi-skimmed milk	+ 235
Salt	No change
Salt-free canned vegetables	+ 85
Sugar	No change
Low calorie drink	+ 130
Syrup-free canned fruit	+ 220
Fruit juice	+ 30

Source: Richardson J. and Grigg J. (1987). Promoting Nutrition Education in Worcester. *Health Education Journal 46*, 25-26.

Information on national and regional trends in food purchase patterns are very helpful in planning further healthier eating promotions. It is also informative to compare changes in your locality with trends elsewhere.

There are a whole series of national agencies, producers, associations and commercial research firms who collect statistics on food production trends and may help you with information. Retail trends in food sales are reported in trade publications which may be consulted in any large library. Most large food processors and retailers have their own marketing departments who may give information if approached. Their addresses may be found on their food packages. Further suggestions on possible sources of information are given in Box 14.2.

Box 14.2

Sources of information on national and regional trends in food production and sales

The following might be willing to supply information if approached:

National Agencies and producers associations
MAFF   Ministry of Agriculture, Fisheries and Food
MLC   Meat and Livestock Commission
NFU   National Farmers Union
The Cocoa, Chocolate and Confectionery Alliance
Potato Marketing Board
Sugar Bureau
Other marketing boards.

Trade publications (describe trends in retail sales)
The Grocer
Hotel and Caterer
Check with the nearest large library for a list of the many trade publications produced.

Marketing departments of food processors	*Retail chains*
Allied Bakeries	Co-op
Rank Hovis MacDougal (RHM)	Tesco
Heinz	Sainsbury
Smedley's	Gateway
Etc., etc.	Safeway
	Etc., etc.

Food sales through caterers

Monitoring food sales is one way of assessing the possible effect of a healthier eating promotion. For example you could look at sales in the hospital staff restaurant before, during and after a promotion in the hospital. The till (cash register) roll can be used to provide information on sales. How much is possible will depend on how sophisticated the till is and the system of accounting used within the catering outlet.

The caterer will first be interested in total sales. They will not welcome any promotion activity which reduces their sales but will be eager to build on and extend any promotion which increases their turnover and profit. This is just as true for institutional caterers as for private sector caterers.

Secondly, you may be able to monitor the sale of specific food items or meals and in some cases the time of purchase. This will give you more idea as to the food choices being made by the customers and whether these are changing. This more detailed monitoring is only possible if the till system records which food items are sold and if the staff using the till are fully aware of the codes to be used when ringing up different purchases.

If mealtimes are staggered within a workplace then time of sale for a food item may be used for identifying differences in food purchasing by different sectors of the workforce. For instance if the shop floor workers' lunch time is 12.00 to 1.00 and white collar workers' lunch time is 1.00 to 2.00, you can compare food preferences and up-take of the promotion messages between different work groups.

Comparative meal sales

Using the till roll system, or knowing the number of meals prepared and sold, you can compare sales of certain food items before, after and during a promotion activity. This information is very useful but may not give you a clear picture of how food purchases are changing. For example are decreased chip sales an indicator that customers are switching to a lower fat form of potatoes source or does it indicate a shift away from all forms of potatoes? Looking at sales of a whole group of products can give you some information on questions such as these. Finding a shift in sales from one food to its healthier alternative is much better evidence of a change in customer purchasing habits than changes in sales of single items.

When consumption of one particular food is reduced (e.g. white bread) there is a tendency for it to be replaced by an alternative food (e.g. wholemeal bread). Similarly a fall in sales of chips during a 'low fat campaign' may be accompanied by a rise in sales of boiled or baked potatoes, pasta and rice. Other examples of alternative foods are shown in Table 14.1.

Table 14.1 Alternative foods for comparative meals sales

Traditional fizzy drinks	Low sugar drinks
Individual portions butter	Individual portions polyunsaturated spread or low fat spread
Meat dishes	Non-meat dishes
Full fat yoghurt	Low fat yoghurt
White bread sandwiches	Wholemeal bread sandwiches
Meat	Poultry, fish

Purchasing contracts

Caterers purchase the food which they prepare and sell from wholesale outlets. Therefore looking back at quantities of raw materials purchased can be helpful. If you wish to evaluate the effect of introducing a district Healthy Eating Policy within a hospital over a year you could look back at purchasing records over three, six or twelve months to note the trends in the purchasing of particular foods. Foods which may be of interest include wholemeal bread, wholemeal flour, white bread, white flour, butter, polyunsaturate-rich margarines and cooking oils, frozen chips, sugar, low sugar drinks and salt.

What is the cause of any changes?

Any changes in purchasing recorded are not necessarily the result of any promotion of healthier eating. (See section on causal inference in Chapter 4.) Other factors which might account for an apparent change are seasonal variation, daily variation in weather conditions, changes in staff, changes in shift systems, changes in the food offered by rival outlets, an advertising campaign on the television, changes in the quality and attractiveness of food, changes in the pricing and marketing of the food or a dozen other factors unrelated to health promotion efforts. Despite this it is usually helpful to know that things have changed even if you are not sure why this has occurred.

Monitoring sales over a long period of time is more reliable than monitoring for a few weeks. Year on year comparisons enable you to rule out seasonal factors or short term variations as a cause.

Before concluding that any improvement (or any deterioration) in food choices is due to health promotion activity think if there is anything else which could have produced it. You may identify events which help the promotion (e.g. marketing drive by the caterer) and you can then build on these. You may also identify things which hinder the promotion (e.g. increased prices of foods you wish to promote) and you can then attempt to remove the barrier.

15 · Data collection in special situations

SECTION A

ASPECTS OF DATA COLLECTION IN SCHOOLS

Introduction

School children and schools are often of special interest in programmes for promoting healthier eating. Eating habits are acquired very young and schools have an important part to play in helping children learn how to choose healthy diets and how to put this knowledge into practice.

When assessing the contribution of schools to healthier eating it is likely that you will wish to consider the following points:

1   What is being taught about health, nutrition and food awareness in the curriculum?
2   What is being served at school meals?
3   What is the tuckshop like?
4   What do the children know and think about food and health?
5   What are the children eating both in school and at home?

It is to be noted that the first three questions are questions mostly about process (what is being done) while the last two are mostly about outcome (what has been achieved).

Seeking permission

The first step in any investigation of food and nutrition in schools is to seek the permission and co-operation of various people. The people to be considered are listed in Table 15.1. The head teacher of the school is a key person and should be able to advise you as to who else should be approached. All the teachers involved in the areas you are investigating will need to be informed and their support solicited. Often you will also have to obtain formal permission from the

215

education authority and maybe from the school governors. Catering staff, other staff and trade unions may also need to be consulted.

Table 15.1   Working in schools – whose permission or help may be needed?

Local Education Authority
Educational advisers
School Governors
Head Teacher
Teachers, heads of departments, class teachers
Catering staff
Other school staff, e.g. classroom assistants
Unions and shop stewards
Pupils
Parents

This seems like a very long list and depending on the type of enquiry you have in mind it may not be necessary to consult all of them. Schools and school catering have recently been subject to a great deal of political controversy and reorganisation. Many of the people whose help you will need may initially be suspicious and it is well worth spending time explaining what you are trying to do and why. Time spent in getting support is never time wasted. Your preliminary discussions are likely to save you from making mistakes and at a later stage people's willingness to co-operate can make all the difference between success and failure.

When you are going to collect information directly from children you must explain to them what information you want and why you want it. Usually you will also have to obtain permission from their parents. What children are eating can be a very sensitive subject and can lead to misunderstandings.

Obtaining parental permission will require special consideration. The usual way is to write a letter explaining what the enquiry is about and asking the parents permission for their child to take part in the study. The letter is often sent home with the child and this is where the problems start. It is well known that many letters entrusted to children are forgotten, lost or mislaid before they reach the parent. Posting the letter may increase the chances of the letter reaching the parent but does not guarantee a reply. Follow-up letters may be no more successful and a personal visit to the home may be needed. Parents of young children who bring their children to or from school can be contacted at the school gate. Sometimes it is possible to call parents to a meeting at which you can explain what you are doing and seek their permission but many parents will not come to meetings. If you are lucky the school may agree to organise obtaining parental permission for you.

216

For some studies it may be reasonable to assume that parents who do not indicate an objection are in agreement. In other studies you will have to exclude from the investigation children whose parents do not positively agree to their taking part.

Curricular activities – what is being taught

It might be sensible to start an enquiry into food and health in schools by looking at what is being taught in the classrooms. The general advisers (called schools' inspectors in some places) in the education authority will be able to explain to you what guidance is given to schools, what specific policies exist and what is actually going on in the different schools in their locality. You can then gather more detailed information from the teachers in a particular school.

Before the introduction of the national curriculum, teaching about food and nutrition could take place under many subject headings. Home economics, biology, physical education, and personal and moral education were usually the main contributors but history, geography, English, mathematics, other sciences and religious education often contributed some teaching on this subject. In primary schools food and nutrition are frequently covered in cross-curricular projects as integrated themes and topics.

With the introduction of the national curriculum there is likely to be less variation in the organisation of subjects within the school. The science and the technology curriculums both specify food and nutrition topics which have to be covered. Even so it will not be possible to appreciate what is being taught in a school without looking at the whole curriculum and identifying the many components relevant to food and nutrition.

Classroom surveys of knowledge and attitudes

The only way to find out what children know about food and health and what they feel about these subjects is to approach them directly. The general principles of knowledge and attitude surveys have been discussed in Chapters 9 and 10. Obviously any instruments must be adapted to the abilities of the age group being investigated. Written methods may be appropriate for older children but for younger children a method which does not involve reading or writing may be needed. For some purposes one to one interviews or group discussions may be the most informative.

There are often opportunities for involving the children themselves in data collection and making the survey into an educational experience. This has the double advantage of providing the school with a learning opportunity and providing you with a large number of data collection assistants. These exercises require careful organisation but can be very worthwhile.

When collecting data in schools usually all the subjects are in the same place and therefore easy to contact. It may also be relatively easy to obtain a high response rate since it is immediately apparent if some children have not responded. On the other hand the situation in which data are collected may produce bias. If the teacher is involved in data collection then the children may give answers that they think will create a favourable impression. Similarly in a group situation they may give answers that will favourably impress their peers or simply imitate the majority. Stressing the confidentiality of any responses and stressing that school authorities will not see replies may help you get unbiased responses.

The ethics of data collection in the school situation have to be considered very carefully. The investigators must satisfy themselves that voluntary informed consent has truly been given and that children are not put under improper pressure to reply.

Eating in the school

Teaching in the classroom about health, nutrition and food is important but what goes on outside the classroom may be even more important in what the child learns. School meals and tuckshops tell us much more about the importance attached by a school to good nutrition than what is taught in home economics, biology or other subjects.

The meals provided by the school are of particular interest. What is on the menu for school lunch? How is it presented and marketed? What are the conditions under which it is served and eaten? What is chosen and how much is left on the plate? What other meals (for example breakfast) are available?

Once again enquiries should start with the education authority:
    Do they have a policy on school meals?
    Are there nutrient specifications or menu guidelines?
    What proportion of pupils take school meals?
    What are the alternatives to eating the school lunch?
    What training is provided for school meals staff?
    Is there a central buying policy?
    Is there a pricing policy to promote sales of any particular foods?
    How much choice is offered? Is it a fixed meal or a cafeteria system?
    What are the budgetary arrangements?

After obtaining answers from the local education authority it is well worth seeking further information at the school level. This may give a rather different picture. Questions to be asked include:
    Is the school dining room pleasant and attractive or is it noisy and dirty with broken furniture?
    What does the menu say?

What foods are placed at the front of the counter? What foods are placed by
the till to stimulate impulse buying?
Are all foods equally available or are some choices sold out in the first five
minutes?
How is the 'lunch hour' organised? Is there time to eat at leisure or are there
competing demands on the children's time?

Simple observation is usually the best way to answer these questions. Half-an-
hour in the school restaurant seeing what goes on will tell you more than reams
of questionnaires. Talking with the children and staff will add further insights
on school meals. Discussion with the catering staff can provide extra useful
information. They may have a different perspective on the subject. What do
they understand by healthy eating and how do they think school meals ought to
be? There may also be hidden factors which while not concerned with nutrition
are vitally important. In one local authority the bonus paid to school cooks used
to depend on how many portions of chips were sold. School cooks may fear that
any change in catering provision could threaten their jobs. It is essential to know
about factors such as these if school meals are to be changed.

The tuck shop

Tuck shops play an important part in school life. The funds they generate are
often important in buying extras which are not funded by the education
authority such as school trips, sports equipment or extra books for the library.
The introduction of LMS (Local Management of Schools) may considerably
increase the pressure on the tuck shop to produce additional funds for the
school. The tuck shop also tells us a great deal about what priority the school
really gives to food and healthy eating. Often the practice in the tuck shop bears
no relation to the theory taught in the classrooms.

The questions to be asked about a tuck shop include:
What items are stocked?
Why are these items stocked? (Ease of storage? Ease of re-ordering and
stocking etc.?)
How are they marketed?
What is the pricing policy? Are profit margins the same on all foods?
What other retailers are competing with the tuck shop for the children's
custom?

Nutritional surveys

Nutritional surveys may be restricted to foods eaten by children at school or they
may consider the children's total food intake. Surveys restricted to foods eaten
at school are much easier to organise but meals eaten at school are only a small
part of a child's overall nutrition (typically about 25% of intake on school

days). In order to understand the full picture you must enquire about the whole day's eating.

The whole range of methods described in Chapters 11, 12 and 13 can be used in a school setting. The fact that all children will be in school for most of the working day can make things easier. Food diaries or records can be collected and checked each day and any queries or ambiguities sorted out while the event is still fresh in the child's memory. Even quite young children can cope with weighed diet records. The school may well make the data collection part of a school activity.

Choosing schools for study

A large education authority may well have several hundred schools and many thousands of school children. Deciding which schools to study deserves careful thought. What type of school do you wish to study? Will you include the schools for children with special educational needs in your study? The education advisers can probably give you a lot of helpful information on the characteristics of the different schools in their locality.

Sampling will probably be a two stage process, first selecting schools and then selecting children (or classes) within schools. Except in very large studies (20 or more schools) random sampling of schools is not advisable. You will do better picking schools (i.e. taking a purposive sample) with the characteristics of interest to you (inner/outer city, urban/rural, ethnic mix, social class mix and so on). The readiness of the staff to co-operate in any data gathering exercise may also be a powerful consideration as to which school you eventually choose.

Further reading

School meals

Birmingham School Meals Working Party (1987). 'Recommendations for school meals.'
Nutrition and Health 4, 237-246.
Wharton B. A. (1987). 'School dinners.'
British Medical Journal 294, 1635.
Community Nutrition Group of British Dietetic Association Information Sheet 14.
Nutritional Guidelines for School Meals.

Schools meals surveys

Bender A. E., Harris M. C. & Getreuer A. (1977). 'Feeding of school children in a London borough.'
British Medical Journal i, 757-759.

McAllister A., Hughes J. & Jones M. (1981). 'A study of Junior School meals in South Glamorgan.'
Journal of Human Nutrition 35, 369-374.

Examples of nutrition surveys in schools
a)   A weighed survey

Nelson M. & Paul A. (1983). 'The nutritive contribution of school dinners and other mid-day meals to the diets of school children.'
Human Nutrition: Applied Nutrition 37A, 128-135.

COMA (1989). *The diets of British school children.*
Report on Health and Social Subject No. 36. HMSO, London.

b)   Food diary

Hackett A. F., Rugg-Gunn A. J. and Appleton D. R. (1983). 'Use of diet diary and interview to estimate the food intake of children.'
Human Nutrition: Applied Nutrition 37A, 293-300.

221

SECTION B

ASPECTS OF DATA COLLECTION IN HOSPITAL

Introduction

Food and nutrition in hospitals may be of special concern for three reasons. First, the hospitals are the 'flagships' of the Health Authorities and may be taken to indicate their corporate values. If healthy eating appears to have left the hospitals untouched then people may reasonably conclude that the Health Authorities think healthy eating unimportant. Second, the hospitals can have a powerful educational effect and each hospital contact represents an opportunity for health promotion. Third, people in hospital are easy and convenient to contact and so hospital studies are a quick way of finding out something about what is happening without mounting a full community survey. Very large numbers of people visit hospitals as outpatients, inpatients or visitors.

The main questions considered in this section are 'Is the hospital promoting healthier eating?' and 'How nutritious and healthy is the usual food served in the hospital?'. It is concerned with the knowledge and attitudes about food and health and the eating behaviour of people in hospital whose dietary requirements are similar to that of the general population. It is not concerned with the assessment of individual intake for clinical purposes nor with special therapeutic diets.

Looking at process – Is the hospital promoting healthier eating?

Hospitals need to look at what they are doing to promote healthier eating. Are there any visible signs of health promotion activity such as posters, or leaflets for staff and patients as one goes round the hospital? Do the menus for patients, the menus in the staff restaurants and the foods in the hospital shop suggest that the hospital is aware of and interested in promotion of healthier eating? Do patients receive advice on eating when they are in the hospital? Do the staff see promotion of healthier eating as a legitimate part of their work? Simple observation will provide an answer to many of these questions. A fuller understanding can be gained by seeking further information from patients and staff in the ways described in the following paragraphs.

Hospital staff

Hospital staff are both targets for health promotion and agents of health promotion. In reality these two roles cannot be separated since unless the staff know about healthier eating and value it for themselves, they cannot be effective in promoting it for their patients.

Enquiries of hospital staff will yield information about how promotion of

222

healthier eating is working in the hospital and how it could be made more effective. Many health districts have laboured to produce a healthier eating policy. Have the hospital staff ever heard of it? Do they know what is in it and could they find a copy if they wished to consult it? Do they feel it has anything to do with them? Do they want to be involved in promotion of healthier eating? Do they feel it is a legitimate part of their job and do they think that their line managers think so? Do they feel they have the time, the resources, the knowledge and the skills to carry out effective promotion of healthier eating? The answers to questions such as these will be vital first in planning health promotion in hospitals and then in monitoring progress and improving programmes.

Asking about staff involvement in promotion of healthier eating leads naturally to asking about their own knowledge and attitudes about healthier eating and their own eating behaviour. This is likely to indicate what training and support staff need in order to become more effective agents for the promotion of healthier eating.

There are many different professional groups in hospital and they all contribute to the functioning of the hospital (Table 15.2). All should feel involved in promotion of healthier eating and a full survey of staff attitudes should consider all staff groups. Each group tends to have its own organisation and lines of communication so you will have to work out the most appropriate way of approaching each one.

Table 15.2   Hospital staff groups

Doctors and medical students

Nurses

Dieticians

Other paramedical professions
(Physiotherapy, O.T., Pharmacy, medical laboratory technicians etc.)

Catering staff

Portering staff

Other hotel services staff

Administration

Clerical staff

What do patients know and think about healthy eating?

Hospitals exist for the benefit of patients and we must seek their views. They can be asked what advice they have received about healthier eating, and whether the advice was interesting, easy to understand, relevant and helpful.

Patients can also be treated as an easily accessible sample of the population of the catchment area. The methods described in Chapters 9 to 13 can be used to assess their knowledge and attitudes about healthier eating and their eating behaviour. Often they will be only too glad to supply this information. Visits to hospital frequently involve long and boring waits so that filling in a questionnaire or being interviewed may seem a pleasant distraction.

Care has to be taken in interpreting information gathered from patients or their visitors because they are not a representative sample of the general population. Some patients such as those with diabetes, hyperlipidaemias or long-standing gastro-intestinal problems may become very knowledgeable about food and health, much more so than the general population. All patients have a health problem and may therefore be especially well informed about things relevant to health and place a higher value on health promotion than other people generally do. Despite these likely biases information gathered from patients and visitors if interpreted with caution can give an indication as to how knowledge and attitudes are shifting in the community.

What patients eat in hospital

The vast majority of patients in hospital have nutritional requirements which are no different from those of normal healthy people outside the hospital. For many of these patients the hospital episode is short and the educational effect of the food served to them in hospital is more important than its nutritional effect.

There will always be an important group of patients who require special therapeutic diets – low calorie, high calorie, low protein, high protein, low salt and so on. This book is not concerned with such patients and ample advice on assessing these diets will be found in textbooks of therapeutic dietetics.

Discussion of hospital food has focused on two main topics. First, does the hospital food supply sufficient energy, protein, vitamins and minerals to meet the needs of normal individuals and the increased need of people recovering from illness? Second, does the hospital food conform to the high fibre, low fat pattern of diet currently advocated?

The first step in looking at what patients eat in hospital is to review the hospital menus. Catering records will show both what choices were available to patients and what choices were made. Examination of plate waste gives an unbiased indication of the quality of the food.

More detailed assessment of the adequacy of hospital catering requires an estimate of the nutrient content of hospital diets and assessment of what patients are eating. Consumption estimates may be rather easier to achieve in a ward setting than when patients are living in their homes. Direct observation of food intake may be relatively easy to arrange. If a standard portion size system is being used in the hospital, quantities of food served may be estimated in this way. Alternatively it may be possible to weigh food as it is served. Plate waste can be noted and weighed as the plates are collected in. Food brought in by relatives and food bought at the hospital shop or trolley must also be noted. This sort of survey is very time consuming but can give an accurate picture of what patients are actually eating.

Long-stay patients

There is a small group of patients in long-stay hospitals for whom hospital food is the only food they get and it is essential that this food should be as healthy and nourishing as possible. Assessment of the diets being eaten on long-stay wards may be particularly rewarding.

An alternative approach to looking at intake is to attempt to assess the nutritional status of patients. Physical signs, anthropometric measures and biochemical and haematological tests can all be used for this purpose (see Box 2.5). Great caution has to be used in interpreting this sort of data since it may be very difficult to distinguish the effects of severe disease from the effects of gross malnourishment (and often the two co-exist). Many articles have been written about this sort of assessment and they will not be discussed further here.

Further reading

Hospital malnutrition

Bender A. E. (1984). 'Institutional malnutrition.'
  British Medical Journal 288, 92-93.
Coates V. (1985).
  Are they being served? Royal College of Nursing, London.

SECTION C

ASPECTS OF DATA COLLECTION IN LARGE EMPLOYERS

Section written by M. Clapham

Introduction

Large employers such as factories, large offices and retailers offer an attractive opportunity for collecting information on populations. It is a convenient way of obtaining information from large groups of healthy people. The organisation of a workplace makes it relatively easy to contact subjects. Before you can collect any data you will need to obtain the permission and support of the employer.

Approaching large employers

When you approach the management of a factory or office the first questions they will ask are 'Why do you wish to collect data?', 'What data do you wish to collect?' and 'What are you going to do with the data when you have collected it?'. You must have your answers to these questions ready prepared.

Remember that commercial organisations exist to make profits, satisfy their customers and provide jobs for their employees. They do not exist to fill in health and life-style questionnaires. They will reasonably ask how helping in your data gathering will benefit them? Possible responses to this question are:
Healthier workforce
Less sickness
Good public relations
Evaluate acceptability of their catering, etc.

Secondly before you attempt to collect data in a large employer you need to understand its management system and philosophy. For example you need to ask 'Who makes decisions? Are they made at national, regional or local level?'. You must get permission from the correct tier of management before you can proceed. Don't forget trade unions and works committees.

Once you have permission then the doors are open for you to start planning data collection. However, in order to succeed you will need to oil the wheels and identify key people at your local level;
Personnel department
Occupational health department
Catering department
Works committee/Trade union group
Health and Safety Committee

One of more of the above groups or individuals may be the key to success and smooth your project through to a satisfactory conclusion. They are particularly likely to be helpful if the data you plan to collect is also useful to them. You may be able to collect some extra data which they want at the same time as you collect data for your own purposes. The adage 'You scratch my back and I will scratch yours!' can be very appropriate.

The personnel and occupational health departments

The personnel or occupational health departments are good places to start planning data collection. Find out what data these departments already have on their workforce such as sex, age, occupation, ethnicity, etc.

From the above information you may decide to collect data on the whole company or to select a target group. You may wish to look at, for example, young males entering the company, or middle management, or blue collar workers eating in the staff dining room, etc.

Ways of monitoring

Once you have decided the group from whom you are going to collect data, i.e. whole workforce or target group, how are you going to do it? First you need to decide the method you wish to use to collect the data, i.e. questionnaires, interviews, suggestion box, etc. Secondly, you need to decide how you are going to make contact with the people from whom you intend to collect data. You will have to make sure that your proposed arrangements are acceptable to the employers and their workforce.

The next paragraphs give a few ideas as to how people can be contacted but it is by no means an exhaustive list.

(a) **Personnel Department**
Employees starting employment or those retiring or leaving the company can be asked to fill in a questionnaire.

(b) **Management/Supervisors**
These can be asked to distribute questionnaires to staff in their section and collect them in again. This can be useful if you wish to gather data on a particular target group within the workforce. This method may also ensure a good completion rate for questionnaires. When a health education initiative has been made with one section of the workforce it may be possible to compare data from them with that from other sections.

(c) **Occupation Health Department**
Occupational health staff can collect data on a routine basis on any member of staff attending their service, particularly if the department offers routine health checks or screening for its employees. This form of data may be useful on a long-term basis and could become part of a pre-employment health screen.

(d) **Unions, Trade Associations, Work Committees, etc.**
These are a useful point of contact. Questionnaires could be distributed by members through their communication systems, i.e. through sections, branches, departments, etc.

(e) **Training courses**
Employees attending any training course can be asked to fill in a health and life-style questionnaire.

(f) **Catering department**
The catering department provides food for the workforce. There are many ways to monitor trends, sales, attitudes, etc., through the catering outlets. These are discussed in Chapter 14.

(g) **Other points of contact**
Wage packet/slips
Changing rooms
Dining rooms/rest areas
Company newsletter
Company magazine
Factory/office entrance
Car park barrier

Summary

There is no substitute for knocking on doors, talking to people about your ideas; what you wish to measure and how you wish to do it. Eventually somebody will listen and let you have a go.

Further reading

Studies with larger employers

Davies L. and Holdsworth M. D. (1985). 'Nutrition and health at retirement age in the United Kingdom.'
Human Nutrition: Applied Nutrition 39A, 315-322.

Rose G. and Shipley M. (1986). 'Plasma cholesterol concentration and death from coronary heart disease: 10-year results of the Whitehall Study.'
British Medical Journal 293, 306-307.

Robert R., Cyster R. and McEwan J. (1988). 'Alcohol consumption and the workplace: Prospects for a change.'
Public Health 102, 463-469.

ASPECTS OF DATA COLLECTION FROM ETHNIC MINORITIES

Introduction

The population of the UK is made up of many different ethnic groups. These include the different groups from the Indian sub-continent, Afro-Caribbeans, different Chinese groups, Malaysians, Vietnamese, Arab, various Eastern European groups and many others. Box 15.1 gives some indication of the size of these groups. These communities have a rich variety of cultures and eating patterns. When collecting data from their members special adaptations to the general methods may be needed.

It is important to avoid the trap of stereotypes. The terms often used, such as 'Asians', 'Afro-Caribbean' and 'Chinese', cover very broad groups and conceal very wide variations among the communities so described. For example, the peoples originating from the different parts of the Indian sub-continent each have their own culture, cuisine and languages and may differ from one another almost as much as they differ from peoples from other parts of the world (see Box 15.2). Similarly each island of the West Indies has its own distinctive characteristics and culture and the different Chinese communities have different customs, cuisine and sometimes language.

All too often we have a preconceived notion of how members of a particular ethnic group will think and behave and this then prevents us from observing what the real situation is. We must always be prepared to collect and examine the data before deciding on the characteristics of any group or member of that group.

Box 15.1

Ethnic groups in England and Wales

	Numbers (thousands)	% UK Born
White	51,107	96
West Indian	534	53
Indian	760	36
Pakistani	397	42
Bangladeshi	103	31
Chinese	115	24
Other	523	–
Not stated	691	–

Source: Social Trends No. 19 Table 1.5.

Box 15.2

Main groups from Indian sub-continent in Britain

Region of origin	Punjab	Gujarat	Pakistan	Bangladesh
Religion	Hindu or Sikh	Hindu or Muslim	Muslim	Muslim
Language	Punjabi	Gujarati	Pakistani	Bengali
Came via E. Africa	Many	Many	Mostly no	Mostly no
Main cereal staple	Chapatti	Chapatti or rice	Chapatti	Rice
Vegetarian	Hindu: most Sikh: some	Hindu: most Muslim: No	No	No
Prohibited meats	Hindu: beef	Hindu: beef Muslim: pork Halal only	Pork Halal only	Pork Halal only
Fish	None	None	Little	Plentiful

Language

Language may make data collection difficult in some situations. Some older members of communities originating from the Indian sub-continent, from the Far East and from parts of Eastern Europe may not be fluent in English. Often a family member will offer to translate questions but this introduces many possibilities for confusion. It is very difficult to be sure whether the answers obtained are those of the respondent, the translator or a mixture of both. Even if the translator is scrupulously accurate the presence of an extra person may alter the responses. Often the translator is a child or grandchild and their relationship with the respondent may affect the replies given.

Translation is particularly hazardous when asking about attitudes. A literal translation may completely alter the meaning of a question, but if the question is freely translated then any pretence at standardisation will be lost.

Some ideas in one culture have no real equivalent in another. Many Asian food systems have ideas of 'hot' and 'cold' foods which are very important in an

230

individual's thinking about food but are difficult to relate to English culture. There is no short cut for cross-cultural interviewing and you have either to go to immense trouble and expense to prepare a properly validated instrument for the group with whom you wish to work (see Box 15.3) or else be prepared to treat any information obtained through a translator with extreme caution.

Box 15.3

Translating a questionnaire for use in another language

1 Start with a questionnaire properly validated in its original language.
2 Discuss the questionnaire with native speakers of the second language.
   Do the questions convey to them the ideas that you wish?
   Are any parts of it likely to be ambiguous or offensive?
3 Get native speakers of the second language to translate your questionnaire into their language.
4 Give the translated questionnaire to another native speaker of the language and get them to translate it back into the original language. Compare this back translation with the original. Where does it differ? Discuss these differences with your translators.
5 When you have a questionnaire which back translates satisfactorily try out the original and translated versions on people who are reasonably fluent in both languages. Do the two versions produce the same responses?
   (Note that these people fluent in two languages will not be representative of the intended target group.)
6 Finally revalidate how the questionnaire works with the intended group.

Religion and culture

Religion is an important element in the beliefs and values of any community. Many religions include dietary proscriptions (see Box 15.4). While there may be a predominant religion for a particular ethnic group it is important to remember that not all members of that group will be adherents of that particular faith and that there may be differences in dietary practice and food beliefs within each religious group.

Different cultures also have different ideas about what is decent and proper. The gender of interviewers has to be considered. In some communities, male interviewers would not be acceptable for female members of the community and equally female interviewers may find it difficult to interview males. Ideas about dress also differ between cultures and standards of dress which would be acceptable for interviews in English culture may not be acceptable in others. There may also be different ideas about cleanliness. For example in some cultures it is polite to remove one's shoes before entering the home.

None of these differences in culture need prevent successful data gathering, but it is important to know what constitutes good manners in the community in which you are working. Carelessness and insensitivity are likely to cause offence and make data collection impossible. Care in observing these conventions will greatly improve the ease and quality of data collection.

Box 15.4

Religious dietary proscriptions

These notes can only be a very rough guide. They attempt to summarise fairly complex rules in a few lines. Furthermore there is considerable variation in the dietary observances among adherents of most faiths.

Hindu
Strictly vegetarian – no meat or fish – beef and pork especially forbidden.
Some may eat eggs.
Alcohol forbidden.
Some periods of fasting.

Muslim
Pork is forbidden – meat must be Halal – slaughtered in a prescribed fashion.
Fish with fins and scales is permitted.
Alcohol forbidden.
Fasting (including no water) observed in daylight hours of month of Ramadan.

Sikh
Orthodox are strict vegetarian – eggs not permitted.
Beef and pork are particularly forbidden.
Alcohol is forbidden.

There is a great deal of variation in dietary observances among Sikh communities.

Jews
Pork is forbidden – meat must be Kosher – slaughtered in a prescribed fashion.
Milk and dairy products must not be eaten at same meal as meat or cooked in same utensils.

Rastafarian
Food must be I-tal.
Meat and eggs may be forbidden.
Salted and canned foods may be forbidden.

Studies of food encounter two problems. First, English food tables are very inadequate for many of the foods eaten in Asian communities. A list of food tables is given in Box 15.5.

Secondly, even when a food is listed in the tables, the values need to be treated with even more caution than usual since there is likely to be very wide variation in the manner in which any particular dish is prepared in different households. It may be possible to circumvent this difficulty by enquiring carefully about the ingredients and cooking methods for each dish and then calculating its nutrient content as described in Chapter 12. This approach is however very time consuming and still involves a great deal of estimation with its attendant errors.

Estimation of portion quantities may also be particularly difficult since many of the dishes are either shared from one pot or else dishes used as garnishes. Under these circumstances it is not only extremely difficult to estimate portion sizes but the content of a portion may differ considerably. Estimates of nutrient intake in members of communities where dishes such as stews, curries and 'soups' figure largely in the diet are likely to be particularly inaccurate.

Box 15.5

Some food tables for ethnic foods

Food composition tables for use in the English Speaking Caribbean (1974). Caribbean Food and Nutrition Institute, Kingston.

Tan S. P., Wenlock R. W. & Buss D. H. (1985). *Immigrant foods*. Second supplement to McCance and Widdowson's the Composition of Foods. Publ. (4th edition) HMSO, London.

Wharton P. A., Eaton P. M. & Day K. C. (1983). Sorrento Asian Food Tables. *Human Nutrition: Applied Nutrition 37A,* 378-402.

Gopalan V., Ramastri B. V. & Balasubramanian S. C. (1976). *Nutritive values of Indian foods*. Hyderabad Institute, National Institute of Nutrition/Indian Council for medical research.

US Department of Health Education & Welfare/FAO. *Food composition tables for use in South East Asia*. FAO, Rome.

Further reading

Henley A. (1980). 'Asians in Britain.'
  Foods and diets. King Edwards Hospital Fund, London.
Fieldhouse P. (1986).
  Food and Nutrition: Customs and Culture. Croom Helm, London.

16 · Presenting the results

by T. Marshall

Summary

The presentation of results must include comprehensible summaries of the data on which the report is founded. The clearest form of data summary is often the graph. More quantitative detail can be included in a table. This chapter outlines how to construct graphs and tables from different sorts of data to illustrate and clarify the inferences drawn from those data.

Introduction

Preceding chapters have explained how quantitative data can be collected. You will then want to explain your findings, draw inferences about the pattern of one variable or the relationship between two variables and possibly make predictions based on your findings. In order to do these things you will need to summarise the data in statistical form. This is also essential before you can communicate your findings to anyone else. It is the aim of this chapter to explain the simpler forms of summarising and presenting numerical data and then how to incorporate them into a report.

Graphs and tables – 'A graph is worth a thousand digits'

Broadly speaking, there are two main forms of presenting data, tables and graphs. Usually it is best to use a mixture of both. A table can contain far more information than a graph, but a graph is usually more readable and more memorable. The eye receives and interprets graphical information 'better' than it does numbers in tables.

There are two main kinds of question to be addressed with statistical methods. The first is 'What is the pattern of...?' which is very much a descriptive question. The second is 'Is there a difference or an association between...?' which is an analytical question.

Neither question considers why the pattern or difference should be as it is. Discussion of 'why' questions requires basic knowledge of nutrition, psychology, education and similar subjects. Chapter 4 described how we attempted to decide whether change could be attributed to health promotion activity. Tables and charts are needed to illustrate and clarify the quantitative basis for these sorts of argument.

Types of data

When deciding how to present results you must remember that the numbers which you have collected are likely to include three different kinds of data or scale. These are nominal, ordinal and ratio (explained in Box 6.2). These different sorts of data have to be handled and presented in different ways.

Figure 16.1 Ways of presenting nominal data

Answers to question 'What was the main dish at last night's meal?'

	Beef/ Veal	Pork	Mutton/ Lamb	Poultry/ Game	Veget- arian	Other	Total
Number	22	29	17	31	11	6	116
Percent	19	25	15	27	9	5	100

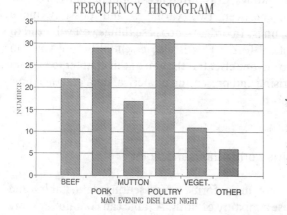

Note that we could draw the histogram either as *absolute* frequencies as here or *relative frequencies* (percentages). What is important is the relative heights of the blocks and this is the same either way round.

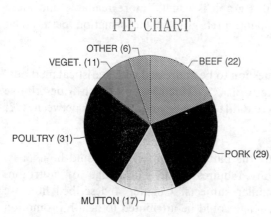

Note that the frequencies are converted to angles which are the appropriate fraction of 360°.

Frequencies and nominal data

We shall begin by restricting attention to the descriptive kind of question, 'What is the pattern of . . . ?'. Suppose we had asked the question:

'What was the main content of last night's meal?' (tick one).
Beef/veal, pork, mutton/lamb, poultry/game, fish, vegetarian, other.

The responses to such a question are nominal data. The best way to present these data is to count up how many responses occur in each category, and to present the totals as percentages, in a table, a barchart or a pie chart (Figure 16.1).

Figure 16.2   Ways of presenting repeated nominal data

The same people are asked the same question about their main meal last night on six occasions. The results can be displayed as follows:

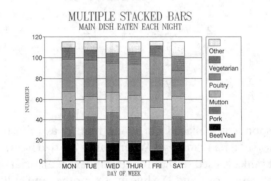

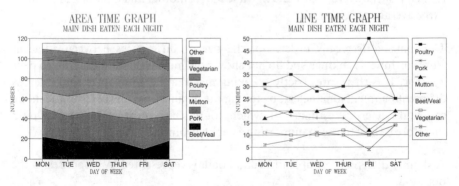

In many ways B and C are clearer, more graphic forms of presentation, but in this example slightly misleading in that:
(i)   they assume equal time intervals between measurements (which may not be the case);
(ii) there is an implicit underlying continuity to the assessments (from having joined up successive time points) which incorrectly invites interpolation.

237

If the question were asked repeatedly on a number of occasions, the results cannot be presented on a single pie-chart and a series of pie charts may be difficult to follow, but a stacked histogram or graph over time may be useful to show change in consumption of particular foods (see Figure 16.2).

Frequencies and ordinal data

Suppose we asked people to rank how much they trusted healthier eating advice from different people. They could be presented with a list of six sources of advice and asked to mark the one they trusted most '1', the second most trusted '2' and so on down to '6' for the least trusted.

If six people are asked to rank the trustworthiness of these sources the table of rankings might look like this:

	A	B	C	D	E	F	Mean rank
			Preference order				
Dietician	1	1	2	1	1	1 = (1.5)	1.3
Own GP	2	2	1	2	2	1 = (1.5)	1.8
Nurse	3	4	3	3	3 = (3.5)	3 = (4)	3.4
Own mother	4	3	4	4	3 = (3.5)	3 = (4)	3.8
Milkman	5	5	6	5	5	3 = (4)	5.0
Politician	6	6	5	6	6	6	5.8

Notice that respondent E placed nurse and mother as joint third trusted and respondent F also had tied rankings. Where ranks are tied like this the average of all the relevant ranks is used so that for respondent F dietician and own GP are ranked 1.5 (the average of 1 and 2) while nurse, mother and milkman are ranked 4 (the average of 3, 4 and 5).

The ranks reflect only order, not the size of differences between adjacent trustworthiness rankings and do not show how much one source is trusted over another. It is therefore strictly speaking meaningless to average ranks across different people. Nonetheless, by taking the mean across all six respondents we can make a crude estimate of which sources are most trusted and would therefore be best to use in supporting a health promotion event.

A slightly different example of ordinal data is represented by responses to the question:

As compared with this time last year are you drinking:
Much more   More   About the same   Less   Much less

There is a true continuity underlying the responses to this question. This sort of data could not sensibly be presented as a pie chart.

Suppose there are two groups of respondents to the question who answer as follows:

	Much more	More	About the same	Less	Much less	Total
Group 1	24	37	32	17	9	119
Group 2	12	17	48	22	19	118

Number of responses in each category

With the trust data the categories had no intrinsic order so we arranged them according to the responses in order of trustworthiness. In the drinking example the categories have an intrinsic order and they must be arranged in this way regardless of how many responses are in each category. 'About the same' comes between 'more' and 'less' even though 'more' is the most popular response in group 1.

Some alternative ways of presenting such data are shown in Figure 16.3. The cumulative distribution (Figures 16.3D and E) show the proportion of the sample with scores 'less than' a given value. If the cumulative distributions are drawn as curves (Figure 16.3E) this implies a truly continuous measurement scale where the 'same' response cover a range extending from very close to 'more' through to very close to 'less' and so on. In judgements of direction of change this is very likely to be the case, though in some ordinal responses continuity may be lacking.

Modal and median responses

We can find the most common, or modal response for any type of data. In the drinking example it was 'more' in group 1 and 'about the same' in group 2. With ordinal scales we can also find the median, the response that divides the entire set of responses into two equal halves. In group 1 there were 119 observations, so that the 60th one in order (from either end) leaves 59 below and 59 above. In group 1, the 60th observation lies in the 'more' category. Where there are an even number of observations (as in group 2 of this example with 118 observations) so that none lies exactly at the middle of the order the median is conventionally estimated as the average of the two observations on either side of the middle' (i.e. the 59th and 60th in group 2). Each of these was in the 'same' category score and so that is the median in group 2.

Ratio scale data

Suppose we have collected some data about the calorie intake of 444 people. It would be possible to write down every individual's intake in a table and you probably did this when examining your results. However, a table of raw data can be a very big table and may make it difficult for you and impossible for other

Figure 16.3 Ways of presenting ordinal data

Answers to question 'As compared to this time last year are you drinking?'

A
Separate
Bar Charts

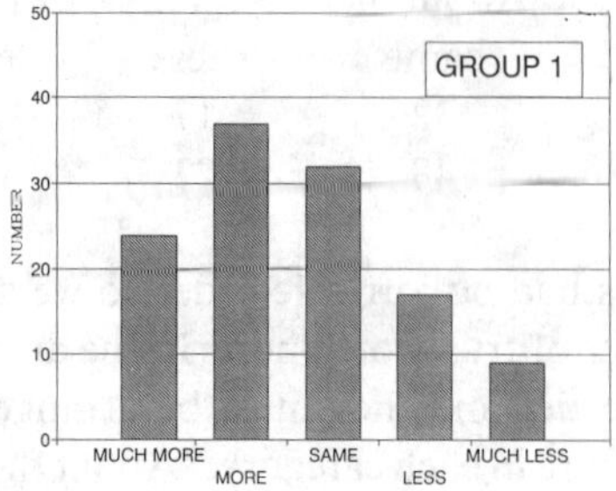

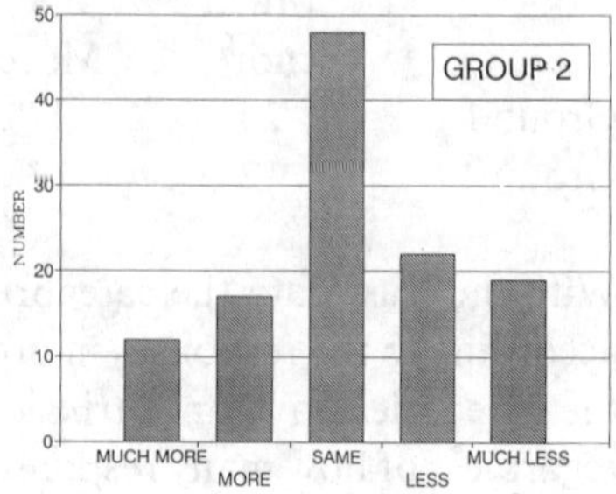

B
Multiple
Bar Charts

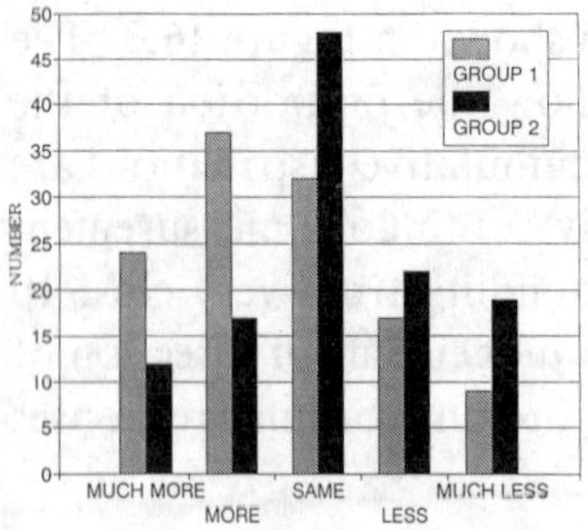

C
Stacked
Bar Charts

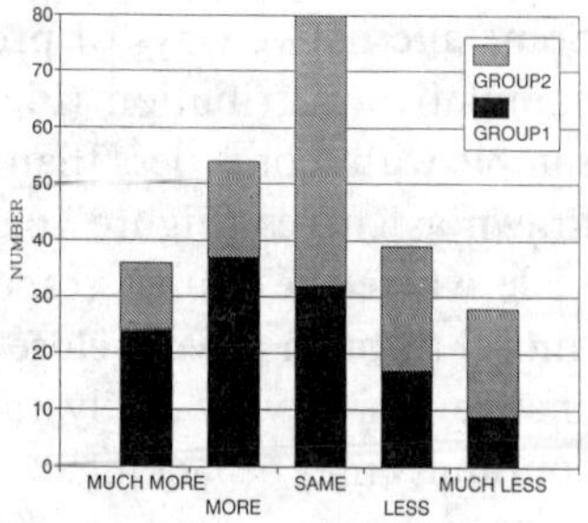

D
Separate
Cumulative
Frequency
Bar Charts

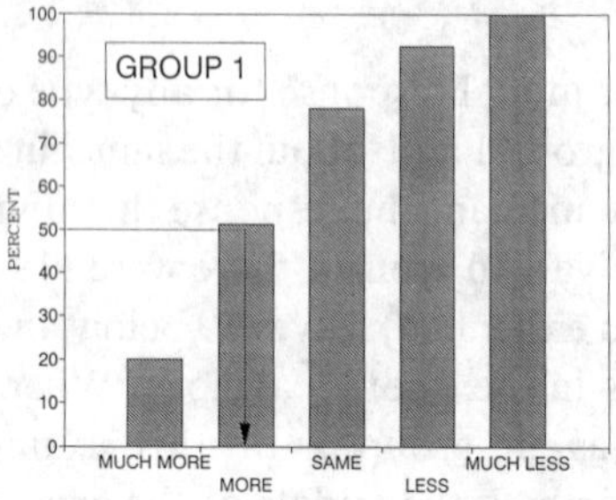

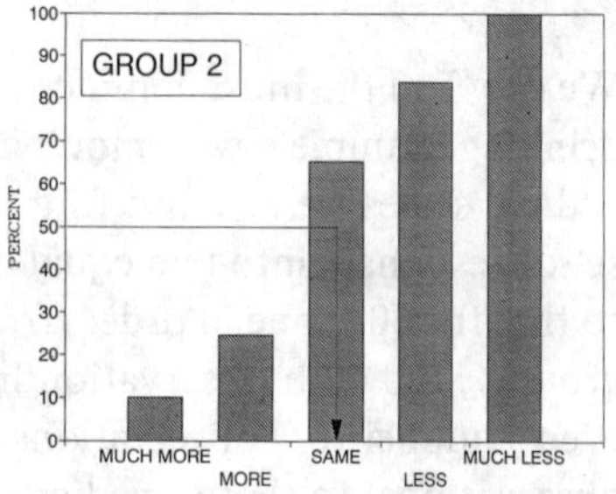

E
Combined
Cumulative
Frequency
Line Plot

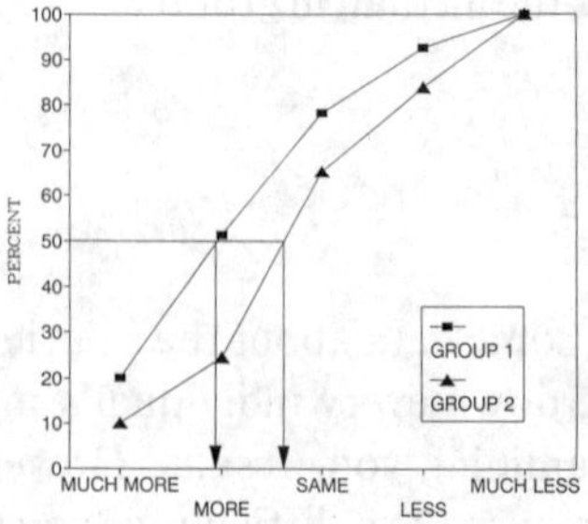

people to see the underlying patterns and trends. Therefore you must summarise the data. A simple way of doing this is a frequency distribution which can then be represented in a table or graphically (see Figure 16.4).

Figure 16.4   Ways of presenting ratio data

Energy intake in a group of 444 people.

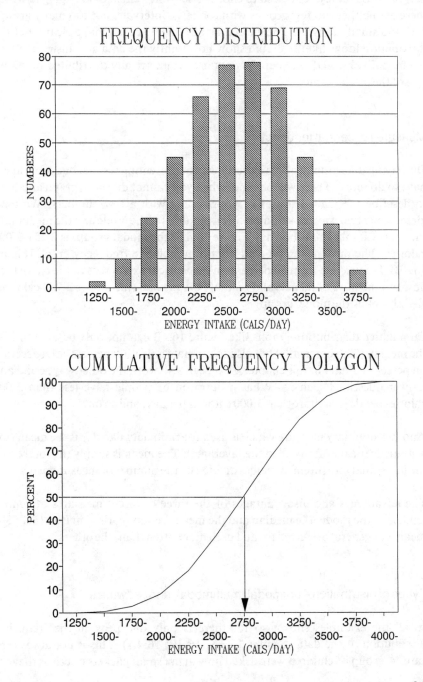

There are several decisions to be taken about combining ratio scale data into groups or bins to create a frequency distribution. How many intervals (bins of data values) should there be? Should they all be the same width? What should be done at the bottom and top of the scale if there are one or two outlying values? Where should the bin boundaries be? Should the intervals be (as in this case) 2,000 to 2,249 cals, 2,250 to 2,499 cals, etc., or 2,001 to 2,250 cals, 2,251 to 2,500 cals, and so on? The answers to these questions will differ according to the nature of the survey. You need to choose a sensible system of grouping in which there are neither too few groups with too large intervals, nor too many groups with too small intervals. The chosen arrangement should make clear what the distribution looks like. It should show how tightly the data are clustered about the modal value and whether the data are symmetrically distributed on either side of the modal value.

Measures of central tendency

Displaying data graphically is a useful way of presenting results, but you usually have to do more. There will be times when you cannot display a graph and have to describe the main features of your results with a few numbers. We have already met two ways of summarising a set of data, the mode and the median. In the energy intake data shown in Figure 16.4A, the modal group, is 2,751-3,000 calories. The median can be read off the cumulative frequency graph (Figure 16.4B). Draw a line from 50 percent on the vertical axis across to the curve then down to the horizontal axis and read off the median (just under 2,750 calories, slightly below the modal group).

Cumulative distribution graphs like Figure 16.4B can not only be used to find the median (50th percentile) but also to estimate any other percentile (see section on percentiles later in this chapter). You can also work the other way round and answer questions such as 'What proportion of people have less than 2,000 calories per day, or more than 3,000 calories per day, and so on?'

Another summary measure which is used for ratio data like this is the mean (the arithmetic mean, often called the 'average'). The mean is simply the total of all the individual measurement values divided by the number of measurements.

The advantages and disadvantages of the three different measures of central tendency, the mode, the median and the mean are summarised in Box 16.1. The mean is in general preferred to, and used more often than, the others.

Types of distribution – unimodal, multimodal, and skewness

In all the examples shown so far there is only one peak in the frequency distribution of the data (Figures 16.3A, 16.3B, 16.4A). This is not always the case. A group of children were asked how many small packets of crisps they ate

242

in the last week and the responses are shown in Figure 16.5A. This is a multimodal distribution. Note that there are several peaks in the response frequency (peaks at 0, 7, and 14 packets). These you will realise correspond to never eating crisps and eating one or two packets a day.

In the calorie consumption example (Figure 16.4A) the calorie intakes were scattered fairly evenly on either side of the median value. This is commonly not the case with nutrient intake data as for example with alcohol intake (Figure 16.5B). Distributions where the response frequency is not evenly distributed on either side of the median are said to be skewed.

The mean is misleading as a description of data sets which are multimodal or strongly skewed and should not be used for them.

Scattergrams

A further way of displaying data can be used where two measurements have been made on the same person (observational unit). The measurement pairs might be weight and age, or serum cholesterol and weight or knowledge of heart disease risk and fat intake. The observational unit could be on an institution such as a Health District or a school rather than a person. For example you might collect the alcohol-related death rate and the per capita expenditure on services for prevention of alcohol-related harm in each Health District.

243

Figure 16.5

	Number of packets of crisps eaten in last week														
	0	1	2	3	4	5	6	7	8	9	10	11	12	13	14<15
Number of children	27	2	1	2	0	5	10	23	4	1	0	2	3	1	12 2

16.5A

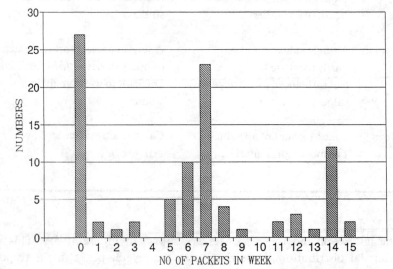

MULTIMODAL DISTRIBUTION
CRISP CONSUMPTION

16.5B

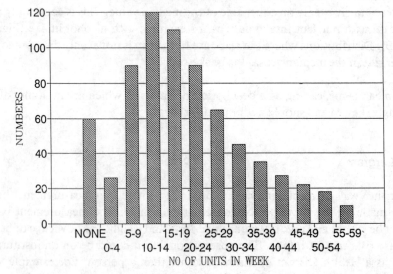

SKEWED DISTRIBUTION
ALCOHOL CONSUMPTION

244

Figure 16.6

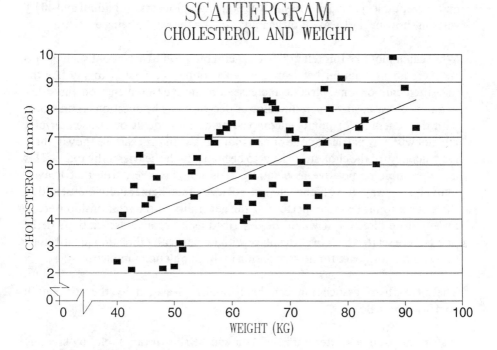

SCATTERGRAM
CHOLESTEROL AND WEIGHT

When data like these are available, the first step is to plot them as a scattergram (Figure 16.6). This diagram allows us to inspect the relationship between the two variables in this set of data.

There are a couple of points to make about such a diagram. Firstly, it is convention that the 'dependent' variable is plotted on the vertical axis and the 'independent' variable on the horizontal axis. What do we mean by 'dependent' and 'independent'? This is sometimes clear, and sometimes less so. For example, it seems reasonable to argue that, to some extent, weight might be dependent upon age (note that this does not mean that age causes a specific level of weight). On the other hand it would be illogical to argue that how old someone was dependent at all on their weight. Therefore age is plotted on the horizontal axis and weight on the vertical axis.

Matters are not always as clear as this, however, as the example of blood cholesterol and weight shows (Figure 16.6). It is easy to argue that your cholesterol level depends on how heavy you are. Yet it is also possible to argue exactly the converse, that how heavy you are depends on your blood cholesterol level or more likely that both weight and cholesterol depend on some third variable. What this example points to is simply that you need to think very carefully before plotting two-variable data.

Secondly, note that the axes of Figure 16.6 are 'broken' between zero and the first measurement on each scale. The reason for this is purely practical: if we didn't do so, the scatter-plot would only occupy the top right-hand corner of the graph, wasting vast areas of graph paper. Breaking the axes in the way shown is quite acceptable, provided you show it. Starting a plot at (say) 3 mmol and 40 kg without showing the breaks is misleading, and on the way to being deceitful.

What can a plot like this tell us? The general question to ask about such data is 'Is there an association between the two variables?'. That is to say 'As the measurements on one variable increase, do the measurements on the other variable increase, stay much the same or decrease?'. The question is concerned with the generality of points encompassing all individuals on the scatter-plot and not with any particular one or two individuals. In the example shown, there is a tendency for the cholesterol level to be higher in the heavier individuals. This is an example of positive association. It is not, however, true that heavier individuals always have higher cholesterol levels than lighter individuals, and so the association is less than perfect. If the generality of the relationship were in the opposite direction it would be described as a negative association. If the points were scattered all over the place with no particular direction identifiable, this would be evidence for no association in the population sampled.

The strength of association can be formally measured by the correlation coefficient (see Box 5.3).

Instead of using a scattergram the data can be shown in a table, by creating group intervals and counting the number of observations falling in each interval. An example of this type of table is shown below:

Cholesterol level	Weight		
	Less than 60 kg	60-79.9 kg	80 kg or more
Less than 6.0 mmol	14	5	0
6.0-6.99 mmol	24	41	16
7.0 mmol and above	3	24	30

In some respects this is a useful summary of the data, and as in the graph you can see the tendency for heavier people to have higher cholesterol levels, and lighter people to have lower cholesterol levels. It is also evident that presenting data like this loses a lot of detail compared with the scatter-plot. Tables such as this are a good way of presenting nominal and ordinal data which might be misinterpreted as continuous variables if presented in a scatter-plot.

Measures of variability

The methods so far presented cover ways of answering the generic question 'What is the pattern of...?' posed at the beginning of this chapter. There is, however, one further concept which is needed to help complete the answer to that question, and that concerns the variability in the sample. Are all the measurements very close together or are they widely scattered?

Three measures of variability are widely available for use with ratio scale data, and they are defined and discussed in Box 16.2. Variability can be measured with nominal and ordinal scale data but that is beyond the scope of this book. The standard deviation (SD) is by far the most commonly used measure of variability for ratio scale data. It is rare to find a mean value in the published literature without also finding a standard deviation attached to it. The standard deviation is a measurement of the amount of variation in the data being described. Where values of any measurement in two groups are compared the data is more widely scattered in the group with the higher standard deviation.

Centiles, quartiles, etc.

The median tells us where the mid-point of the data lies that is to say the point below which 50% of the observations fall. We can describe the distribution further by stating the points below which 25% (one quarter) and 75% (three quarters) of the observations fall; these divisions are called quartiles. We can describe the distribution further by stating the points below which 10% (10th percentile) and 90% (90th percentile) fall and so on. It was explained earlier how cumulative frequency graphs (Figure 16.4B) can be used to find these points.

Box 16.2

Measures of variability for ratio scale variables

For explanation of terms used in the mathematical expressions see footnote.

Name	Definition	Comments
Range	The biggest measurement minus the smallest measurement.	Easy to calculate. Unreliable because it depends totally on extreme values.
Semi-interquartile range	[75th percentile value minus 25th percentile value], divided by two.	Easy to calculate (though it may depend on the accuracy of a graph). Difficult to use with further analytical methods.

Continued overleaf

Box 16.2 Continued

Standard deviation

$$\sqrt{\frac{\Sigma (X - \bar{x})^2}{(N - 1)}}$$

Moderately difficult to calculate (but can often be done automatically by pocket calculators and computer packages).

This equivalent expression is often more convenient for use in calculations.

Calculation of SD is very important in further analytical work.

$$\sqrt{\frac{\Sigma X^2 - (\Sigma X)^2 / N}{N - 1}}$$

Measures of error of mean

Two other measures are related to the standard deviation. They are not measures of variability but measures of the likely error attached to your estimate of the mean.

Standard error of mean (SEM)

$$\frac{SD}{\sqrt{N}}$$

You can be 95% sure that the mean lies within ±2 SEMs of the value given.

95% confidence limit $t \times SEM$

Another way of showing how sure you are about the value given for the mean.

Explanation of mathematical terms used:

X   is the values of the measurement

$\bar{x}$ is the mean

Σ indicates the sum of i.e ΣX is all the values of X added together.

t   depends on sample size and confidence level. For 95% confidence limit t is approximately 1.96 provided sample size is not very small.

Reporting results of analytic studies

Many studies will include analytic aims of the kind exemplified in the following questions:

1 Is there a difference in the frequency of second heart attack between those given dietary advice after their first heart attack advice and those not given advice?
2 Is there an association between body weight and serum cholesterol?
3 Is there a difference in knowledge of coronary heart disease risk factors between those people who received a booklet and those who did not?
4 Are levels of knowledge about fat and heart disease associated with lower consumpton of fat in the diet?

Analytic studies of this type require you to present your results in a way that supports statistical inferences. For example you will have to argue whether apparent differences or associations in the samples you studied are evidence for differences or associations in the populations from which they were drawn. It is essential to note that statistical analysis does not answer questions about the cause of any difference or association that may be found. Those questions require consideration of the study design (discussed in Chapter 4) and also of broader scientific issues.

You should have thought about how you will use the data to draw inferences before they were ever collected and long before the data analysis or report writing stage. This book cannot describe the complete range of statistical and other methods available for analysing data though a few hints can be given. Unless you are sure how data will be used to draw inferences it is imperative that you consult an expert at the design stage of a study – not at the end of data collection. No statistician likes being approached by someone with a lot of data to analyse, when no contact has been made previously. All too often nothing useful can be done. A famous statistician once remarked that the best that can usually be done in such circumstances is to give the data a decent burial.

Testing for differences between groups

Statistical methods can help to measure the reality of apparent difference in proportions or mean values between groups by assessing their significance in statistical terms. For example, a statistical test will tell you how likely it is that you would have obtained a particular set of results if there were really no difference between groups.

Suppose a study was mounted to answer the first question about the effect of dietary advice on risk of repeated heart attacks. The results are that of the 70 patients who received dietary advice 11 had second attacks whereas of the 60 who did not receive advice (control) 21 had second attacks. A statistical test will tell us that if the two groups come from populations with the same risk the probability of getting a difference as big as this is between 1 in 20 and 1 in 100. (This is an example of testing the null hypothesis – see Box 3.3.) We can infer that the apparent difference in risk of second attack between groups is probably real and that if the groups were comparable in all other respects that receiving of dietary advice has made a difference.

Testing for associations between variables

Similarly, with respect to the second question, on body weight and cholesterol, a cloud of points as in Figure 16.6 suggests that higher body weight is associated with higher cholesterol. If the cloud of points had sloped in the other direction that would suggest a higher cholesterol was associated with lower body weight. A statistical test will tell us how likely we would be to get a cloud with that shape and apparent direction if there were really no association (null hypothesis). Another statistical test can measure the strength of the association. We can derive formulae from the data that enable us to predict someone's cholesterol if we know their body weight, and we can calculate how big the errors in these predictions are likely to be.

There is a wide range of statistical methods for summarising data, using them to test hypotheses and drawing out underlying trends. Sadly the wrong answers can easily be obtained and wrong conclusions be drawn if the wrong methods are used or the right calculations wrongly interpreted. Guidance is therefore needed, both with respect to what questions to ask and what statistical procedures to use. Books are far from being the solution for all problems, but they may be useful if there is no local statistical expertise available and you have a basic idea of how to proceed. Some useful titles are given at the end of the chapter.

If there is a single message to be obtained from this section it is that analysis and interpretation of the results, and that includes the simple graphical presentation of them depend critically on study design. Design and analysis should not (and indeed, cannot) be regarded as separate activities. They are intrinsically part of the same whole, and should be recognised as such before embarking on a study in the first place.

Presenting results honestly

Reports must give enough information for people to see how you arrived at your conclusion and for them to see if they agree with your interpretation. Suppose someone else did a study intended to answer our first question about the effect of dietary advice on risk of repeat heart attacks. They proudly report the outcome that 11% in the dietary advice group and 33% in the other group had second attacks. This might sound impressive, until you find out that there were only nine subjects in each group. The difference (a three-fold difference!) is the consequence of only two subjects responding differently (1 out of 9 in the advice group and 3 out of 9 in the other group). Presenting the results in percentage terms while strictly true was grossly misleading. If there had been more patients (say 90) in each group we might have been able to say something worthwhile about the results. With only 9 in each group the most that could be said about the results is that it might be worth doing a proper study.

This study was fatally flawed from the beginning. Had they sought proper statistical advice they would have realised that if a difference as big as 10% against 30% really existed between the treatment groups they would have needed about 50 in each group in order to have an 80% chance of demonstrating it. (Box 7.12 shows a similar problem.)

And now some words

Research and surveys are a waste of time unless they are written up in a way that is understandable and convincing. Now you have thoroughly examined your data, you have thought about what they mean and how they should be interpreted and you have summarised them in a series of attractive graphs and tables. It only remains to assemble them into a useful report.

This may either be presented by oral report at a workshop, seminar or conference or by written report. An oral presentation (talk) has to be different in style from a written report. You usually have to be very selective concentrating on your main conclusions with the evidence that supports them.

It is very helpful to use a few visual aids but these should be simple and well designed. Avoid the temptation to cram detailed tables, or multiple graphs onto an overhead or slide. If people want to know the mechanics of your study or particular details they will ask you questions afterwards and you should have replies for these prepared in readiness.

Written presentation

The first thing to establish is what sort of report is required. Occasionally several hundred pages with many appendices and masses of detail may be appropriate. More often five or ten sides of A4 is required and sometimes just a single side of paper. Frequently different types of report have to be prepared for different people; maybe a fairly long and detailed report for your immediate manager and a much shorter one for those less directly concerned with your results. The length and style of the report has to be appropriate both for its intended readership and for its contents.

A full report should begin with a short summary which highlights the conclusions and the evidence for them. The key graphs and tables which support your conclusions will form the skeleton of a report. They will need to be fleshed out with a short written explanation of what they show and what conclusions you draw from it. It is usually helpful to begin the report with a short statement of why the study was undertaken and what questions you intended to answer. Longer reports will also include sections on the methods to collect the data and a summary of what was already known about the subject to put the results in context.

Improving readability

It is worth spending some time on the presentation of the report since this makes it much easier to understand and increases the likelihood that it will be read and acted on. Modern word processing packages and photocopiers make it relatively easy to produce quite professional-looking reports with more than one typeface (fonts). Check that the report is laid out nicely with adequate space left between sections and not too many words squashed onto the page. Make generous use of sub-headings. If possible get graphs and tables close to the words which describe them so that the reader can easily skip from text to graph and back again.

There are other devices that you can use to bring your report to life. Selective quotes can add a lot to a report. A quote such as 'thought the hospital cooking was delicious – best he had eaten for years' adds colour in a way that a pie chart showing that 76% rated the cooking as good or very good cannot. (The report 'Healthy eating on a low income', published by HEA, is a very good example of the illustrative use of selected quotes.) Photographs added to a report can greatly enhance its interest but are usually too awkward and expensive to reproduce.

Usually you have to resist the urge to include a lot of supporting detail. Sometimes it can be added as an appendix so that it is available to those who want it but does not clutter up the main text. Often it is better simply to note that the material is available and say how those who want it can obtain it from you.

The whole purpose of preparing a report is to communicate your findings to others. The suggestions in this section are intended to help you produce the sort of report that people find easy and pleasurable to read. A clear, concise, well-presented report is a key tool in persuading people to act upon your findings.

Further reading

Some useful statistical books for the uninitiated

Anderson A. J. B. (1989). *Interpreting Data*. Clapham and Hall, London.

Kirkwood B. (1988). *Essentials of Medical Statistics* (8th edition). Blackwell Scientific, Oxford.

Statistics at Square One by T. D. V. Swinscow – British Medical Association, London, 1983.

Presentation skills

British Medical Association (1985). *Presenting a paper. How to do it – 1*. (2nd edition). British Medical Association, London.

Printed in the United Kingdom for HMSO
Dd294059 1/92 C15 G3390 10170